Liver Disease

Stanley Martin Cohen
Perica Davitkov

Editors

Liver Disease

A Clinical Casebook

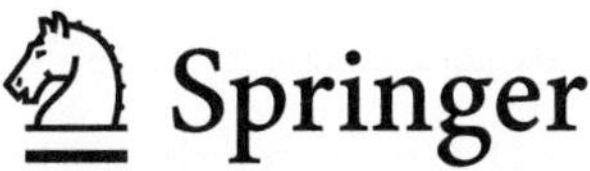 Springer

Editors
Stanley Martin Cohen
Case Western Reserve University
School of Medicine
University Hospitals of Cleveland
Cleveland
OH, USA

Perica Davitkov
Case Western Reserve University
University Hospitals of Cleveland
Cleveland
OH, USA

ISBN 978-3-319-98505-3   ISBN 978-3-319-98506-0   (eBook)
https://doi.org/10.1007/978-3-319-98506-0

Library of Congress Control Number: 2018963224

This Springer imprint is published by the registered company Springer Nature Switzerland AG
The registered company address is: Gewerbestrasse 11, 6330 Cham, Switzerland

Preface

The field of clinical hepatology has been rapidly advancing over the last several years. Much of this has been fueled by the extraordinary developments and treatments for viral hepatitis (especially hepatitis C). However, extensive research into all aspects of liver disease has provided significant insights and therapeutic developments and opportunities in a variety of liver-related conditions.

Liver disease is a common and often confusing medical issue that is frequently encountered in general clinical practice. There are a multitude of clinical manifestations seen with liver disease, especially in those patients with cirrhosis and portal hypertension. Because of this, caring for patients with liver disease can be somewhat overwhelming to the general care provider. Our goal with this book is to provide a systematic and logical approach to the diagnosis and treatment of patients with a variety of liver conditions.

In this clinical casebook, we have put together case-based presentations to go through a number of common clinical scenarios seen in patients with liver disease. The chapters each present a case and then pose a number of clinically relevant questions. The authors then answer the questions as a mechanism to describe the various liver conditions. Figures and tables have also been incorporated into the text to enhance the educational experience.

As the editors (as well as chapter authors) of this manuscript, we have had the honor and privilege of working with a large group of world-renowned authorities in the field of liver disease. Many of the chapter authors are leaders in their field and have been instrumental in developing the current, international diagnostic and therapeutic guidelines. In addition, many of them are world-renowned researchers in the field of liver disease. We wish to acknowledge each and every one of the authors for their hard work. This book would not have been possible without their considerable time and effort.

We also wish to thank the publishers for their editorial and overall support.

Finally, we hope that this book provides the reader with a comprehensive review of liver disease and that it will serve as a valuable resource for providers caring for patients with liver disease.

Cleveland, OH, USA   Stanley Martin Cohen
                                                         Perica Davitkov

Contents

Contributors

Joseph Ahn Department of Medicine, Division of Gastroenterology and Hepatology, Oregon Health and Science University, Portland, OR, USA

Naim Alkhouri University of Texas Health San Antonio, Department of Gastroenterology, San Antonio, TX, USA

Texas Liver Institute, San Antonio, TX, USA

Yumi Ando Department of Medicine, Division of Gastroenterology and Hepatology, Oregon Health and Science University, Portland, OR, USA

Lydia Aye Division of Gastroenterology and Hepatology, Loma Linda University, Loma Linda, CA, USA

Jason J. Cano Division of Gastroenterology and Hepatology, Baylor College of Medicine, Houston, TX, USA

Kristina R. Chacko Division of Gastroenterology and Liver Diseases, Department of Medicine, Montefiore Medical Center, Albert Einstein College of Medicine, Bronx, NY, USA

Stanley Martin Cohen Hepatology, Digestive Health Institute, University Hospitals Cleveland Medical Center, Cleveland, OH, USA

Division of Gastroenterology and Liver Disease, Case Western Reserve University School of Medicine, Cleveland, OH, USA

Melissa Corson Departments of Medicine, University of California at Los Angeles, Los Angeles, CA, USA

Thomas Couri Department of Internal Medicine, University of Chicago Medical Center, Chicago, IL, USA

Perica Davitkov Louis Stokes VA Medical Center, Cleveland, OH, USA

Case Western Reserve University, Cleveland, OH, USA

Digestive Health Institute, University Hospitals Cleveland Medical Center, Cleveland, OH, USA

Yngve Falck-Ytter Louis Stokes VA Medical Center, Cleveland, OH, USA

Case Western Reserve University, Cleveland, OH, USA

Digestive Health Institute, University Hospitals Cleveland Medical Center, Cleveland, OH, USA

Guadalupe Garcia-Tsao Section of Digestive Diseases, Yale University School of Medicine, New Haven, CT, USA

Section of Digestive Diseases, VA CT Healthcare System, West Haven, CT, USA

Nael N. Haddad University of Texas Health San Antonio, Department of Internal Medicine, San Antonio, TX, USA

Mona Hassan Department of Gastroenterology and Liver Disease, Henry Ford Hospital, Detroit, MI, USA

Sofia Simona Jakab Section of Digestive Diseases, Yale University School of Medicine, New Haven, CT, USA

Section of Digestive Diseases, VA CT Healthcare System, West Haven, CT, USA

Eric Kallwitz Division of Hepatology, Department of Medicine, Loyola University Chicago Stritch School of Medicine, Maywood, IL, USA

Daniel B. Karb University Hospitals, Cleveland, OH, USA

Paul Y. Kwo Stanford University School of Medicine, Palo Alto, CA, USA

Cynthia Levy Division of Hepatology, University of Miami Miller School of Medicine, Miami, FL, USA

Joseph K. Lim Section of Digestive Diseases, Yale University School of Medicine, New Haven, CT, USA

Zurabi Lominadze Division of Gastroenterology and Nutrition, Department of Medicine, Loyola University Chicago Stritch School of Medicine, Maywood, IL, USA

Mazyar Malakouti University of Texas Health San Antonio, Department of Gastroenterology, San Antonio, TX, USA

Arthur McCullough Lerner College of Medicine at Case Western Reserve University, Cleveland, OH, USA

Lindsay Meurer University Hospitals Cleveland Medical, Center Case Western Reserve University, Cleveland, OH, USA

Dilip Moonka Medical Director of Liver Transplantation, Division of Gastroenterology and Liver Disease, Henry Ford Hospital, Detroit, MI, USA

Lisa M. Najarian Departments of Surgery, University of California at Los Angeles, Los Angeles, CA, USA

Stephen C. Pappas Division of Gastroenterology and Hepatology, Baylor College of Medicine, Houston, TX, USA

Raj Mohan Paspulati Digestive Health Institute, Head of GI and GYN Radiology, Division of Abdominal Imaging, Department of Radiology, University Hospitals, Case Western Reserve University, Cleveland, OH, USA

Anjana Pillai Division of Gastroenterology, Hepatology, and Nutrition, University of Chicago Medical Center, Chicago, IL, USA

Anthony Post Division of Gastroenterology and Liver Disease, University Hospitals Cleveland Medical Center, Case Western Reserve University, Cleveland, OH, USA

John F. Reinus Division of Gastroenterology and Liver Diseases, Department of Medicine, Montefiore Medical Center, Albert Einstein College of Medicine, Bronx, NY, USA

Mark W. Russo Carolinas Medical Center, Charlotte, NC, USA

Sammy Saab Departments of Medicine, University of California at Los Angeles, Los Angeles, CA, USA

Departments of Surgery, University of California at Los Angeles, Los Angeles, CA, USA

Sasan Sakiani Department of Gastroenterology and Hepatology, Digestive Disease Institute, Cleveland Clinic, Cleveland, OH, USA

Andrew R. Scheinberg Department of Internal Medicine, University of Miami Miller School of Medicine/Jackson Memorial Hospital, Miami, FL, USA

Paul A. Schmeltzer Department of Hepatology, Carolinas Medical Center, Charlotte, NC, USA

Seth N. Sclair Division of Gastroenterology and Liver Disease, University Hospitals Cleveland Medical Center, Case Western Reserve University School of Medicine, Cleveland, OH, USA

Shivani Ketan Shah Yale Traditional Internal Medicine Residency, New Haven, CT, USA

Dennis L. Shung Section of Digestive Diseases, Department of Medicine, Yale-New Haven Hospital, New Haven, CT, USA

Marina G. Silveira Yale School of Medicine, New Haven, CT, USA

Amandeep Singh Cleveland Clinic, Department of Gastroenterology and Hepatology, Cleveland, OH, USA

Tram Tran South Bay Gastroenterology, Torrance, CA, USA

Katherine Wong Stanford University School of Medicine, Palo Alto, CA, USA

Chapter 1
Drug-Induced Liver Injury

Dennis L. Shung and Joseph K. Lim

Introduction

Drug-induced liver injury (DILI) accounts for about 50% of acute liver failure cases in the United States. Diagnosis is challenging, especially due to the myriad combinations of potentially hepatotoxic medications and clinical presentations. Unexplained liver injury should prompt a thorough investigation of medication administration (e.g., for accidental or intentional overdose) and the use of herbal and dietary supplements. The framework for approaching DILI includes the following: (1) categorize the injury as either intrinsic or idiosyncratic, (2) establish time course and pattern of injury, and (3) triage effectively to minimize mortality risk.

D. L. Shung
Section of Digestive Diseases, Department of Medicine,
Yale-New Haven Hospital, New Haven, CT, USA
e-mail: dennis.shung@yale.edu

J. K. Lim (✉)
Section of Digestive Diseases, Yale University School of Medicine,
New Haven, CT, USA
e-mail: joseph.lim@yale.edu

© Springer Nature Switzerland AG 2019
S. M. Cohen, P. Davitkov (eds.), *Liver Disease*,
https://doi.org/10.1007/978-3-319-98506-0_1

Clinical Case Scenario

A 75-year-old gentleman presented to his primary care physician with malaise and jaundice for several days. He has a history of hypertension, hyperlipidemia, and osteoarthritis. He had several joint surgeries in the past, primarily of the shoulder and knee. He takes atorvastatin, amlodipine, and as-needed Tylenol and ibuprofen. He had recently seen a homeopathic practitioner who had recommended taking silver therapy. Family history reveals no known history of liver disease or autoimmune disease. He denied tobacco, alcohol, or illicit drug use. He is married, is a retired former realtor, and has one adult son. His physical exam is notable for scleral icterus and mild tenderness in the right upper quadrant. He was alert and fully oriented, with no asterixis and no hyperreflexia. He has no stigmata of chronic liver disease. Initial labs revealed ALT 5169 U/L, AST 4494 U/L, alkaline phosphatase 70 U/L, total bilirubin 3.1 mg/dL, direct bilirubin 2.7 mg/dL, INR 1.4, and albumin 4.5 g/dL. CBC and kidney function were within normal limits.

Questions

1. What features would you use to triage the patient, and how would you risk stratify his liver injury?
2. Which medications are common culprits (especially in this case), and how do you differentiate DILI from other etiologies?
3. What are the patterns of liver injury and how do they relate to DILI?
4. What are the treatment options for this patient's presumed DILI?
5. When should a liver biopsy be obtained?

Discussion

Question 1. What features would you use to triage the patient, and how would you risk stratify his liver injury?

This patient presents with acute liver injury. It is important to differentiate acute liver injury from acute liver failure (ALF), since the latter requires emergent evaluation for transplantation. First determine if this is indeed a de novo liver injury with no previous signs of hepatic impairment (<26 weeks). Then, assess for signs of neurologic failure (asterixis, decreased mental status or confusion), multiorgan failure, and degree of coagulopathy (INR >1.5).

Dr. Hyman Zimmerman made the observation that patients with hepatocellular DILI and jaundice had high mortality of 10–40%. This has become known as "Hy's law." Furthermore, MELD score and coma grade on admission are the strong predictors of the need for liver transplantation, although prognostic scores are somewhat poor or rudimentary. Due to the extremely poor prognosis of ALF from DILI, liver transplantation may provide a rescue.

Question 2. Which medications are common culprits (especially in this case), and how do you differentiate DILI from other etiologies?

Exposure to known hepatotoxic medications should not preclude a thorough evaluation for other causes of acute liver injury since DILI remains a diagnosis of exclusion. These include acute ischemic hepatitis, malignancy with infiltration, Budd-Chiari syndrome, heatstroke, Wilson's disease (serum ceruloplasmin), acute hepatitis B (HBsAg and anti-HBcIgM), acute hepatitis A (HAV-IgM), and hemochromatosis (iron level, transferrin saturation, and ferritin). If epidemiologically relevant, consider hepatitis E, hepatitis D coinfection, HSV, VZV, or EBV. Review for toxic exposures including Amanita mushroom poisoning. Less common but important diagnoses include autoimmune hepatitis and alpha-1-antitrypsin deficiency (ANA, anti-mitochondrial antibody, anti-LKM1, IgG levels, and alpha-1-antitrypsin phenotype).

When evaluating this patient, it is important to obtain a clear history of medication use including prescription medications, over-the-counter agents, and herbal supplements. In our patient, he is using acetaminophen as well as silver therapy, and he could be at risk for both intrinsic and idiosyncratic DILI. Intrinsic DILI is predictably dose-dependent and most commonly caused by acetaminophen, which our patient takes "as needed" for joint pain. With excessive acetaminophen use, labs would be expected to show extremely high aminotransferase elevation (>3500 IU/L). On biopsy, acetaminophen-induced liver injury would be expected to show a predominant centrilobular hepatocyte injury. As little as 3–4 gm/day of acetaminophen can cause acute liver injury (especially in patients using significant amounts of alcohol), although most ingestions have >10 gm/day. Idiosyncratic DILI has a less consistent relationship to dose and varies in its presentation depending on susceptibility of individuals. Other homeopathic remedies in this case are of particular concern, specifically silver, which in susceptible individuals can cause DILI.

Usually hepatotoxic drug reactions are characterized by rapid onset of malaise and jaundice, but each has its own pattern of injury (hepatocellular, cholestatic, or both). Allergic reaction are generally absent except in sulfa drugs (fever, rash, eosinophilia) and phenytoin (fever, lymphadenopathy, rash), and 20% of severe liver injury cases are idiosyncratic reactions.

Age and gender can also be associated with different susceptibility for DILI; in this patient's case, increased age can increase the risk of DILI from isoniazid, amoxicillin-clavulanate, and nitrofurantoin. For children, Reye's syndrome caused by aspirin-, valproate-, and propylthiouracil-induced liver injury is more common. Women appear to be at higher risk to have a DILI that appears as a chronic hepatitis resembling autoimmune hepatitis with minocycline, methyldopa, diclofenac, nitrofurantoin, and nevirapine. Environmental (smoking, EtOH, infection/inflammation) and drug-related risk factors (dosage, metabolic profile, class effect/cross-sensitization, and polypharmacy) can also predispose a patient to idiosyncratic DILI.

A multitude of herbal remedies have been associated with DILI including germander, chaparral leaf, and usnic acid. Though statins have been associated with transient aminotransferase elevations, acute toxicity is rare. Livertox.nih.gov is a helpful website to look up the prevalence of drug-related liver injury for specific agents.

Question 3. What are the patterns of liver injury and how do they relate to DILI?

Usually, DILI occurs within the first 6 months of taking a new medication, although the latency can be variable. The R-value is the serum alanine aminotransferase/upper limit of normal (ULN) divided by alkaline phosphatase/ULN. R > 5 is considered hepatocellular, R < 2 cholestatic, and 2–5 "mixed." Hepatocellular liver injury refers to a predominant abnormality in aminotransferase levels. Aminotransferases include AST and ALT that are enzymes that transfer amino groups of aspartate and alanine to ketoglutaric acid. ALT is primarily present in the liver, while AST is present in cardiac and skeletal muscle, kidney, and brain tissue.

Cholestatic liver injury is characterized by a predominant abnormality in alkaline phosphatase and total and direct bilirubin. Alkaline phosphatase is a zinc metalloproteinase enzyme that catalyzes phosphate ester hydrolysis and is found in the canalicular membrane of the hepatocyte (not bile duct) as well as the bone, placenta, intestine, and kidney. It increases when bile ducts are obstructed due to increased canalicular synthesis and translocation to the sinusoid, but the other canalicular enzyme GGT can be used to confirm that the elevation is from the liver. Bilirubin is predominantly in its unconjugated form (indirect) and becomes conjugated by UDP-glucuronosyltransferase to direct bilirubin that allows excretion into bile. Conjugated bilirubin elevations are present in both hepatocellular and cholestatic disorders due to impairment in bile flow but can be helpful for diagnosing significant obstruction. Elevation in indirect bilirubin is likely from another process, most commonly hemolysis.

See Table 1.1 for several medications and herbal products that can cause DILI, their latency period, and their typical pattern of liver injury.

Table 1.1 from Chalasani et al. AJG 2014 provides a breakdown of typical liver injury patterns

Medication	Latency	Typical pattern of injury/identifying features
Antibiotics		
Amoxicillin/ clavulanate	Short to moderate	Cholestatic injury (but can be hepatocellular), DILI onset frequently detected after cessation
Isoniazid	Moderate to long	Acute hepatocellular injury (similar to viral hepatitis)
Trimethoprim/ sulfamethoxazole	Short to moderate	Cholestatic injury (but can be hepatocellular)
Fluoroquinolones	Short	Variable
Macrolides	Short	Hepatocellular (but can be cholestatic)
Nitrofurantoin		
Acute form (rare)	Short	Hepatocellular
Chronic form	Moderate to long	Typical hepatocellular; resembles idiopathic autoimmune hepatitis
Minocycline	Moderate to long	Hepatocellular
Anti-epileptics		
Phenytoin	Short to moderate	Variable with immune-allergic features (fever, eosinophilia)
Carbamazepine	Moderate	Variable with immune-allergic features
Lamotrigine	Moderate	Hepatocellular with immune-allergic features
Valproate		
Hyperammonemia	Moderate to long	Elevated blood ammonia, encephalopathy

Table 1.1 (continued)

Hepatocellular	Moderate to long	Hepatocellular
Reyes-like syndrome	Moderate	Hepatocellular, acidosis
Analgesics		
Nonsteroidal anti-inflammatory agents	Moderate to long	Hepatocellular
Immune modulators		
Interferon-beta	Moderate to long	Hepatocellular
Interferon-alpha	Moderate	Hepatocellular; resembles autoimmune hepatitis
Anti-TNF agents	Moderate to long	Hepatocellular; resembles autoimmune hepatitis
Azathioprine	Moderate to long	Variable, can have portal hypertension due to VOD and NRH
Herbals and dietary supplements		
Green tea extract (catechin)	Short to moderate	Hepatocellular
Anabolic steroids	Moderate to long	Cholestatic
Pyrrolizidine alkaloids	Moderate to long	SOS/VOD
Flavocoxid	Short to moderate	Mixed
Miscellaneous		
Methotrexate (oral)	Long	Fatty liver, fibrosis
Allopurinol	Short to moderate	Variable, granulomas with immune-allergic features
Androgen-containing steroids	Moderate to long	Variable
Inhaled anesthetics	Moderate to long	Cholestatic
Inhaled anesthetics	Short	Hepatocellular
Sulfasalazine	Short to moderate	Variable
Proton pump inhibitors	Short	Hepatocellular; very rare

Question 4. What are the treatment options for this patient's presumed DILI?

There are no specific therapies or antidotes for the majority of drug-induced liver injury cases; the cornerstone is withdrawal of the offending medication. For acetaminophen, N-acetylcysteine (NAC) repletes glutathione, which is depleted after lipophilic drugs have been conjugated to glutathione and excreted into the kidney or GI tract. It is most effective within 1 h of ingestion, can be beneficial 3–4 h after ingestion, and can even be considered up to 48 h after ingestion. For non-acetaminophen early-stage ALF, NAC should be considered due to some evidence for improved transplant-free survival in early coma grade patients (52% with NAC vs 30% with placebo). Surprisingly, children should not receive NAC due to one trial demonstrating a lower rate of 1-year survival.

Overall, supportive care with antihistamines for symptomatic pruritus while undergoing a "washout" or "de-challenge" period can help elucidate the diagnosis. Typically, cholestatic DILI patterns usually take longer (up to 180 days) than hepatocellular DILI (60 days) to resolve.

Afterward, monitoring for chronic DILI (15–20% of cases) should be pursued to document complete resolution, particularly for patients with cholestatic liver injury.

Question 5: When should a liver biopsy be obtained?

Overall, for drug-induced liver injury, liver biopsy has low diagnostic yield. If the etiology is unclear, a biopsy can be considered specifically if you suspect an acute episode of autoimmune hepatitis with negative autoantibodies or there is a previous history of cancer. However, if aminotransferases are persistently elevated despite cessation of potential culprit medications, a biopsy would be more helpful. Reasonable timeframes to consider liver biopsy include 60 days for predominantly hepatocellular liver injury and 180 days for predominantly cholestatic injury. Of note, a biopsy can also differentiate between viral infection and metabolic disease (e.g., Wilson's disease).

Patient Treatment Course

After obtaining a thorough history, the patient reported starting the silver therapy but self-discontinuing after 2 to 3 days due to progressive symptoms. He was taking high doses of acetaminophen, up to 10 extra-strength (500 mg) tablets daily due to worsening joint pain. His last dose of acetaminophen was the day prior to his visit. He was admitted to the inpatient ward and received NAC. His AST and ALT normalized rapidly with no long-term sequelae.

Conclusions

Drug-induced liver injury is an uncommon but important cause of acute liver injury and can lead to acute liver failure requiring transplantation. The most important clinical tools are obtaining a thorough history, excluding other causes of liver injury, withdrawing the offending agent, and providing supportive care including N-acetylcysteine. While idiosyncratic drug-induced liver injury has a wide variation in its presentation and outcome, the majority improve with cessation of the offending agent.

Further Reading

1. Chalasani NP, et al. ACG clinical guideline: the diagnosis and management of idiosyncratic drug-induced liver injury. Am J Gastroenterol. 2014;109:950–66.
2. Kwo PY, Cohen SM, Lim JK. ACG practice guideline: evaluation of abnormal liver chemistries. Am J Gastroenterol. 2017;112(1):18–35.
3. Lee WM. Drug-induced hepatotoxicity. NEJM. 2003;349:474–85.
4. Lee WM, Stravitz RT, Larson AM. Revised American Association for the Study of Liver Diseases position paper on acute liver failure. Hepatology. 2012;55(3):965–7.
5. Reuben A, Koch DG, Lee WM. Drug-induced acute liver failure: results of a U.S. multicenter, prospective study. Hepatology. 2010;52:2065–76.
6. Stravitz RT, et al. Autoimmune acute liver failure: proposed clinical and histological criteria. Hepatology. 2011;53:517–26.

Chapter 2
Acute Alcoholic Hepatitis

Sasan Sakiani and Arthur McCullough

Introduction

Alcohol-induced liver disease is the leading cause of chronic liver disease worldwide and remains the second most common cause of cirrhosis in the United States. Heavy alcohol use, which is defined by more than three drinks per day for men and more than two drinks per day for women for over 5 years, can lead to a broad range of chronic liver diseases, including steatosis (60–100% of patients), steatohepatitis and fibrosis (20–40% of patients), and eventually cirrhosis (10–20% of patients) and hepatocellular carcinoma (3–10%). Acute alcoholic hepatitis (AH) is a clinical diagnosis that is based on the development of jaundice and hepatocellular injury that occurs in 35–40% of patients with heavy alcohol use and has been associated with 20–50% mortality in untreated patients. In this chapter, we describe a case of a patient presenting with severe AH. We discuss diagnosis, prognosis, treatment options, and outcomes.

S. Sakiani
Department of Gastroenterology and Hepatology, Digestive Disease Institute, Cleveland Clinic, Cleveland, OH, USA

A. McCullough (✉)
Lerner College of Medicine at Case Western Reserve University, Cleveland, OH, USA
e-mail: mcculla@ccf.org

© Springer Nature Switzerland AG 2019

S. M. Cohen, P. Davitkov (eds.), *Liver Disease*,
https://doi.org/10.1007/978-3-319-98506-0_2

Clinical Case Scenario

A 54-year-old male presents to the emergency room with a 1-week history of progressive jaundice and abdominal distention. He has a history of hypertension and arthritis. He denied any history of surgery. He takes occasional naproxen for chronic low back pain; otherwise he is not taking any over-the-counter, herbal products or prescribed medications. He typically drinks four to five beers per day after work and occasionally more on the weekends. He smokes half a pack a day. He has never had a blood transfusion. He denies any tattoos. He did experiment with IV drugs 30 years ago. He is married with two children and works as an accountant. His vital signs are BP 110/57, HR 105, RR 15, and temperature 36.7. His physical exam reveals significant jaundice and scleral icterus. He has multiple spider angiomas on his upper chest and back and a distended abdomen with protruding flanks. Labs performed in the emergency room reveal:

- ALT: 60 U/L
- AST: 130 U/L
- Alkaline phosphatase: 150 U/L
- Total bilirubin: 12 mg/dL
- Albumin 3.4 g/dL
- INR: 1.8
- Platelets: 95
- Hemoglobin 11.2
- MCV: 105
- Creatinine: 1.1 mg/dL
- Sodium: 134 mmol/L
- Hepatitis C antibody: negative
- Hepatitis B surface antigen: negative
- Hepatitis B surface antibody: positive
- Hepatitis A surface antibody: negative
- Antinuclear antibody (ANA): negative
- Smooth muscle antibody (SMA): negative

A right upper quadrant ultrasound shows a slightly enlarged liver with coarsened echotexture. The gallbladder is unremarkable and there is no biliary dilation. There is also moderate ascites present within the abdomen.

He is admitted to the hepatology service for further management.

Questions

1. How is the diagnosis of acute alcoholic hepatitis made?
2. What is the prognosis of this patient?
3. What are treatment options for this patient?
4. Is liver transplantation an option for this patient?

Discussion

Question 1. How is the diagnosis of acute alcoholic hepatitis made?

The diagnosis of AH is mainly based on clinical presentation. Patients typically present with new or worsening jaundice in the setting of chronic, heavy alcohol use up to 8 weeks prior to presentation. This should not be confused with alcoholic steatohepatitis, which is the presence of fatty liver plus hepatic inflammation and fibrosis seen in patients with chronic excessive alcohol intake. However, AH can occur in any stage of alcoholic liver disease and 80% of patients presenting with AH may have underlying cirrhosis and thus can present with other complications of cirrhosis and sepsis.

Patients often present with non-specific symptoms such as fatigue, right upper quadrant abdominal pain, or loss of appetite along with new or worsening jaundice (see Table 2.1). Patients are often malnourished and may have evidence of sarcopenia. Other signs of chronic alcohol use and underlying advanced liver disease and portal hypertension may also be present, including spider angiomas, palmar erythema, splenomegaly, ascites, and hepatic encephalopathy. Hepatic encephalopathy should not be confused with alcohol withdrawal, which usually

Table 2.1 Signs and symptoms of alcoholic hepatitis

Nausea/vomiting
Abdominal pain (usually right upper quadrant and/or midepigastric)
Weakness
Anorexia
Malnourishment
Jaundice
Fatigue
Fever
Increased abdominal girth with ascites
Tender hepatomegaly
Hepatic encephalopathy
Bruit heard over the liver
Variceal bleeding

Stigmata of chronic liver disease
  Spider angiomata
  Palmar erythema
  Gynecomastia
  Parotid enlargement
  Increased venous collaterals across the anterior abdominal wall
  Dupuytren's contractures

involves more agitation, tremors, tachycardia, and even seizures. The presence of systemic inflammatory response syndrome (SIRS) features is also common and warrants investigation for potential sources of infection.

Laboratory findings in patients with AH include serum total bilirubin of greater than 3 mg/dL along with transaminases elevated greater than 1.5 times the upper limit of normal but usually less than 400 U/L. The AST to ALT ratio of greater than 1.5 helps differentiate this from other causes of hepatitis, although other causes of liver disease including biliary disease and drug-induced liver injury need to be ruled out. Although patients with AH often present with leukocytosis in the absence of infection, it is important to investigate all potential infectious etiologies. Serum albumin is often low and can be due to malnutrition, inflammation, or the severity of the underlying liver disease. The INR can be elevated on presentation for similar reasons. BUN can also be low in patients with chronic alcohol use but can be elevated in patients presenting with renal failure or GI bleed. Other laboratory abnormalities include elevated serum creatinine, hyponatremia, hypokalemia, and hypomagnesemia.

The 2018 guidelines by the American College of Gastroenterology (ACG) have proposed three definitions and subtypes of AH:

1. *Definite* AH, in which there is histological confirmation of features of AH in a patient with a compatible clinical diagnosis
2. *Probable* AH, which is a clinical diagnosis based on heavy alcohol use for more than 5 years along with active alcohol use until 4 weeks prior to presentation, sudden onset or worsening of jaundice, AST/ALT ratio more than 1.5:1 with levels <400 IU/L, and the absence of other causes of liver disease
3. *Possible* AH, where the clinical diagnosis is uncertain due to another confounding etiology or unclear history of alcohol use

Patients presenting with possible AH may benefit from a liver biopsy to confirm the diagnosis. The characteristic histologic findings on a liver biopsy include macro-vesicular steatosis, ballooned hepatocytes, Mallory-Denk bodies, lobular infiltration of neutrophils, cholestasis, and fibrosis, which is often pericellular and sinusoidal. It is important to note that these findings are similar to those in nonalcoholic steatohepatitis (NASH), and thus the patient's history and other laboratory findings, such as those listed previously, may be helpful in distinguishing between the two. Also, as mentioned previously, many patients with AH may have underlying advanced liver disease or cirrhosis, and in these cases some of the features such as steatosis may not be prominent. When performing a liver biopsy, the transjugular approach is preferred given the increased risk of bleeding as well as the inability of patients to comply during a percutaneous liver biopsy.

Our patient has a clinical history and presentation that is typical for AH and thus he has probable AH. The ultrasound does not show any evidence of biliary disease, although it does show some evidence of underlying cirrhosis. Other common causes of liver disease such as viral hepatitis, autoimmune hepatitis, and drug-induced liver injury have been ruled out as well. Therefore, a decision was made that he does not require a liver biopsy.

Question 2. What is the prognosis of this patient?

Depending on the severity, AH can have a mortality as high as 65%. The severity and prognosis typically depend on the number of organs systems involved and the underlying degree of liver disease. In addition, the degree of malnutrition plays a very important role in prognosis, with one study demonstrating mortality rates up to 80% in veterans with severe malnutrition. Having other concomitant diseases such as hepatitis C (HCV) or obesity also affect the prognosis, with one study demonstrating 20–25% higher mortality in those with concomitant HCV. As previously mentioned, up to 80% of patients who present with AH already have underlying cirrhosis, and those who are obese are two times more likely to have cirrhosis than nonobese individuals.

Several scoring systems have been used to help predict AH mortality, and many of these have demonstrated good predictive values for 30-day mortality (see Table 2.2). Unfortunately, they are less accurate for predicting mortality at 90-days or longer, as abstinence from alcohol remains the key factor for long-term survival. The most commonly used scoring system is the Maddrey discriminant function (MDF), which involves a calculation involving prothrombin time (PT) and total bilirubin. A score of ≥32 is associated with a 30-day mortality of 20–50% and has thus been used for initiating treatment with corticosteroids in patients with severe AH. However, the MDF relies on PT, for which normal values vary across different laboratories and is thus not universally consistent. On the other hand, the

Table 2.2 Prognostic clinical scoring systems for alcoholic hepatitis

Scoring system	Calculation formula	Severe disease indicator
Maddrey discriminant function	4.6 × [patient's prothrombin time (seconds) – control prothrombin time (seconds)] + bilirubin (mg/dL)	≥ 32
MELD (model for end-stage liver disease)	$3.8 \times \log_e$ bilirubin (mg/dL) + $11.2 \times \log_e$ INR + $9.6 \times \log e$ creatinine (mg/dL) + 6.4	≥ 20
Glasgow alcoholic hepatitis score	Age < 50–1 point Age ≥ 50–2 points	≥ 9
	WBC < 15 K – 1 point WBC ≥ 15 K – 2 points	
	Urea <5 mmol/L – 1 point Urea ≥5 mmol/L – 2 points	
	INR < 1.5–1 point INR 1.5–2 – 2 points INR > 2–3 points	
	Bilirubin <125 μmol/L – 1 point Bilirubin 125–250 μmol/L – 2 points Bilirubin >250 μmol/L – 3 points	
	The total score is the sum of the above factors	
ABIC (age, bilirubin, INR, creatinine)	Age (years) × 0.1 + bilirubin (mg/dL) × 0.08 + creatinine (mg/dL) × 0.3 + INR × 0.8	> 9
Lille score	Calculator available at www.lillemodel.com	> 0.45

model of end-stage liver disease score (MELD), which has been shown to be comparable to the MDF in predicting 30-day mortality, uses INR rather than PT, making it consistent across laboratories. A score ≥ 20 has been associated with 20% mortality at 90 days. The MELD score has the added benefit of being used for liver transplant listing and has become increasingly utilized in prognosticating AH.

Other scoring systems include the ABIC (age, bilirubin, INR, and creatinine) score, the Glasgow score, and the Lille score. The ABIC score is similar to the MELD score with the addition of age as a variable and has been shown to be comparable to the MDF and MELD. The Glasgow score utilizes age, WBC, urea, INR, and bilirubin and may also be useful to determining which patients benefit from the use of corticosteroids, although it is not widely utilized in the United States. The Lille score, which uses age, albumin, creatinine, PT, and bilirubin at days 1 and 4 (originally day 7), has been shown to predict response to corticosteroids when the score is less than 0.45. In addition, the combination of MELD at baseline and Lille score has been shown to be the most effective for predicting 2-month and 6-month mortality.

In addition to these scoring systems, other biomarkers such as serum lipopolysaccharide levels and SIRS criteria are helpful in predicting mortality. In particular, the presence of SIRS criteria on admission predisposes to acute kidney injury and the development of hepatorenal syndrome, as well as multi-organ failure.

Our patient has a MELD score of 25 and an MDF greater than 32. Using these criteria, our patient has severe AH with at least 20% mortality at 30 and 90 days and may benefit from corticosteroids.

Question 3. What are treatment options for this patient?

While mild cases of AH often improve with supportive care, treatment options for AH remain limited, with long-term mortality in severe AH remaining as high as 30–40% despite treatment. Patients with severe AH should be admitted with the initiation of general supportive care measures as well as for the work-up for underlying infectious etiologies, particularly if SIRS criteria are present. For hypotensive patients, volume replacement with albumin is generally preferred over crystalloids.

As previously mentioned, many of these patients are malnourished on presentation. As such, nutritional support has been the mainstay of treatment with many randomized controlled studies demonstrating some improvement in survival with enteral or parenteral supplementation. Patients with severe AH require daily protein intake of 1.2–1.5 g/kg with a caloric intake of 35 Kcal/kg. In addition, patients may require replacement of thiamine, B complex vitamins, and other minerals such as zinc, magnesium, and potassium.

Options for pharmacologic therapy are limited with conflicting findings in various studies. The most studied medications include corticosteroids (prednisolone) and pentoxifylline. The landmark STOPAH (steroids or pentoxifylline for alcoholic hepatitis) study, which was the largest randomized placebo-controlled multicenter study, demonstrated a trend for mortality benefit at 28 days with prednisolone compared to placebo, with an odds ratio of 0.72 (95% CI, 0.52 to 1.01; $p = 0.06$). However, there was no improvement in outcomes at 90 days or 1 year. As noted in the previous section, a Lille score calculated at day 4 or 7 of <0.45 predicts response to corticosteroids, and these patients should complete a 28-day course of prednisolone (40 mg daily). However, those with scores >0.45 should discontinue prednisolone. It is important to note that corticosteroids increase the risk of infectious complications (13% vs 7% in placebo during the STOPAH trial) and work-up for underlying infections should be performed before initiating treatment and monitored during treatment. In addition, the use of corticosteroids is relatively contraindicated in patients who present with gastrointestinal bleeding.

Pentoxifylline, which is a phosphodiesterase inhibitor, did not show any survival benefit in the STOPAH trial. However, prior studies have demonstrated that pentoxifylline can reduce the risk of hepatorenal syndrome by up to 53% and can thus be considered for this purpose. Studies have not shown any improvement in outcomes with the combination of pentoxifylline and corticosteroids, or as salvage to corticosteroid failures.

While N-acetylcysteine (NAC) is typically felt to improve outcomes in drug-induced liver injury (particularly acetaminophen-induced), a study has demonstrated short-term (1–2 months) survival benefit when NAC was used in combination with prednisolone. Unfortunately, as with other treatment options, this benefit did not extend to long-term (6-month) survival.

Other treatment options that are being studied and which may eventually be helpful in the treatment of severe AH include granulocyte colony-stimulating factor (G-CSF), Anakinra (IL-1 receptor antagonist), antibiotics, obeticholic acid, fecal transplants, and extracorporeal liver support systems such as the molecular adsorbent recycling system (MARS).

It is important to remember that the key to long-term survival remains complete abstinence of alcohol, and thus all patients should be referred to alcohol rehabilitation centers and counseling early in the clinical course.

Our patient was started on tube feeds through a Corpak in addition to receiving thiamine and folate supplementation and was placed on a CIWA protocol to monitor for alcohol withdrawal. He was also given vitamin K 10 mg subcutaneously to see if his INR would improve. Prednisolone 40 mg by mouth daily was started after work-up for infectious etiologies, including a diagnostic paracentesis, chest X-ray, urinalysis, and blood cultures which were all unremarkable. On day 7 of treatment, his labs reveal total bilirubin 17 mg/dL, AST 125 U/L, ALT 57 U/L, creatinine 1.5 mg/dL, INR 2.1, and sodium 134 mmol/L.

The Lille score at day 7 is 0.521 (>0.45), which predicts a poor prognosis and non-response to corticosteroids. Prednisolone is thus discontinued. The patient and his family are now asking about other treatment options.

Question 4. Is liver transplant an option for this patient?

Historically, patients with alcoholic liver disease are not referred for transplant evaluation at the same rates as those with other causes of liver disease. Also, while UNOS does not list it as a requirement, many transplant programs have incorporated a 6-month abstinence rule, where patients with alcoholic liver disease are required to show complete abstinence from alcohol and participation in alcohol rehabilitation programs. The purpose of this rule is to identify patients who are at increased risk of recidivism and to allow time for potential recovery and improvement in liver function, which is often seen in the first 6 months after cessation from alcohol. Unfortunately, given the high mortality rates in patients with severe AH, many of these patients are unable to qualify for liver transplant or become too sick for transplant before completing the 6-month rule. In addition, until recently, many programs considered AH an absolute contraindication for liver transplant despite data showing good outcomes. For example, a study from France demonstrated that carefully selected patients who underwent liver transplantation for severe AH did better than those who did not (77% vs 23% survival at 6 months, $p = 0.001$) and had an overall 2 year survival rate of 71%, which is comparable to other forms of liver disease, while a subsequent study demonstrated an even greater survival benefit (89% vs 11%, $p < 0.001$) at 6 months.

Given these and other studies demonstrating similar findings, more centers are now transplanting patients for severe AH without waiting for the 6-month rule as long as they meet other criteria such as no prior episodes of AH, never previously being told by a physician that alcohol intake was causing liver damage, and having good psychosocial support at home. Other predictors of recidivism include younger age, underlying psychiatric disorders, longer duration of alcohol abuse, higher amounts of alcohol abuse, polysubstance abuse, and prior failed rehabilitation attempts. Careful selection of patients undergoing liver transplantation for AH is important to minimize the risk of recidivism which can potentially lead to failure of the allograft.

As in all patients undergoing evaluation for liver transplantation, work-up for other comorbidities is essential. Patients with alcoholic liver disease are particularly at increased risk for cardiovascular comorbidities, such as dilated cardiomyopathy and hypertension. Chronic alcohol abuse has also been associated with other comorbidities including malnutrition, chronic kidney disease, dementia, psychiatric disorders, and the use of cigarettes and/or recreational drugs. Patients undergoing liver transplant for AH are also at increased risk for de novo malignancy compared to other causes of liver disease, with studies showing rates that are 2 to 3 times higher than in nonalcoholic liver disease transplant recipients, particularly in those who smoke cigarettes.

Given that our patient failed corticosteroid therapy and is worsening based on rising bilirubin, INR, and creatinine, he may benefit from liver transplantation. The fact that this was his first episode and that he was never told previously that his drinking was contributing to his liver disease is a good prognostic indicator. In addition, prior to admission he appears to be high-functioning with a job and good family support. He was referred for transplant evaluation and was determined to be a low-risk for recidivism by a psychiatric evaluation. He was still referred to AA meetings which he started to attend 3 times per week after discharge. After completing his evaluation, he was discussed in the transplant selection committee and was unanimously accepted to be listed for transplant with a MELD score of 31.

Conclusions

AH occurs in patients with chronic heavy alcohol use and can occur at any stage of alcoholic liver disease. It is a clinical diagnosis involving new or worsening jaundice with bilirubin typically greater than 3, along with elevated AST and ALT (less than 400 U/L) with AST:ALT ratio greater than 1.5:1. Liver biopsy is rarely necessary to make the diagnosis unless there is an atypical presentation or there are competing etiologies for liver disease such as herbal or medication use. AH can range from mild cases requiring supportive care alone to severe cases which can have up to 20–65% mortality despite treatment. Several scoring systems can be used to help predict severe AH and an increased risk of mortality, including the MDF ($\geq$32) and MELD score ($\geq$20). All patients should be given routine supportive measures including nutritional support. Unfortunately, pharmacological treatment options are limited, particularly for long-term survival. Corticosteroids (prednisolone) have been shown to improve short-term mortality rates and can be used after ruling out underlying infections or GI bleeding, although they are also associated with increased risks of infectious complications. The Lille score may be used for determining non-response to corticosteroids and in combination with the MELD score is helpful in predicting 6-month mortality. Finally, liver transplantation should not be withheld in patients with severe AH who fail corticosteroid therapy as it has been shown to improve survival with low rates of recidivism in carefully selected patients, with long-term outcomes comparable to other causes of liver disease.

Further Reading

1. Drinane MC, Shah VH. Alcoholic hepatitis: diagnosis and prognosis. Clin Liver Dis. 2013;2(2):80–3.
2. Garcia-Saenz-de-Sicilia M, Duvoor C, Altamirano J, Chavez-Araujo R, Prado V, de Lourdes C-MA, et al. A Day-4 Lille model predicts response to corticosteroids and mortality in severe alcoholic hepatitis. Am J Gastroenterol. 2017;112(2):306–15.
3. Lucey MR. Liver transplantation for alcoholic liver disease. Nat Rev Gastroenterol Hepatol. 2014;11(5):300–7.
4. Mathurin P, Moreno C, Samuel D, Dumortier J, Salleron J, Durand F, et al. Early liver transplantation for severe alcoholic hepatitis. N Engl J Med. 2011;365(19):1790–800.
5. Mendenhall C, Roselle GA, Gartside P, Moritz T. Relationship of protein calorie malnutrition to alcoholic liver disease: a reexamination of data from two veterans administration cooperative studies. Alcohol Clin Exp Res. 1995;19(3):635–41.

6. Singal AK, Bataller R, Ahn J, Kamath PS, Shah VH. ACG clinical guideline: alcoholic liver disease. Am J Gastroenterol. 2018;113(2):175–94.
7. Thursz MR, Richardson P, Allison M, Austin A, Bowers M, Day CP, et al. Prednisolone or pentoxifylline for alcoholic hepatitis. N Engl J Med. 2015;372(17):1619–28.

Chapter 3
Ascites

Ascites in Cirrhosis

Melissa Corson, Lisa M. Najarian, and Sammy Saab

Introduction

Ascites is often the index presentation of decompensation in patients with cirrhosis. The presence of ascites is an important cause of morbidity and mortality as well as healthcare utilization. The treatment of ascites revolves around the combination of lifestyle changes, diuretic therapy, and, in severe cases, more invasive techniques. In this chapter, we describe the evaluation

M. Corson
Departments of Medicine, University of California at Los Angeles,
Los Angeles, CA, USA

L. M. Najarian
Departments of Surgery, University of California at Los Angeles,
Los Angeles, CA, USA

S. Saab (✉)
Departments of Medicine, University of California at Los Angeles,
Los Angeles, CA, USA

Departments of Surgery, University of California at Los Angeles,
Los Angeles, CA, USA
e-mail: ssaab@mednet.ucla.edu

© Springer Nature Switzerland AG 2019
S. M. Cohen, P. Davitkov (eds.), *Liver Disease*,
https://doi.org/10.1007/978-3-319-98506-0_3

and management of a patient with new-onset ascites. We also highlight the differential diagnosis of ascites.

Clinical Case Scenario

A 68-year-old male presents to his primary care doctor for several weeks of worsening abdominal fullness and fatigue. He has a diagnosis of hypercholesterolemia and diabetes mellitus type 2. He denies a past history of surgery. His medications include metformin and atorvastatin. Upon further questioning he admits to drinking several cases of beer a week for the past 40 years. He denies smoking or illicit drug use. Vital signs are within normal limits. The physical examination is significant for palmar erythema, spider angiomata on his chest, a nodular liver edge, and shifting dullness on his abdominal exam. His labs are significant for thrombocytopenia of 125×10^3/microliter and an elevated international normalized ratio (INR) of 1.4.

You are concerned that he has new-onset ascites and order a formal abdominal ultrasound that confirms your suspicion.

Questions

1. How is the diagnosis of ascites made? What is utility of abdominal ultrasound in diagnosis of ascites?
2. Once a diagnosis of ascites is made, how does one determine the cause of ascites? What is the differential diagnosis?
3. What is the management of ascites? What are the options once a patient fails to respond to initial medical management?

Discussion

Question 1. How is the diagnosis of ascites made? What is utility of abdominal ultrasound in diagnosis of ascites?

It is important to be able to diagnose ascites in both the inpatient and outpatient setting as it may be the first clinical manifestation of cirrhosis. The four main physical signs of ascites are bulging flanks, flank dullness, shifting dullness, and a fluid wave. If a clinician notices a full, bulging abdomen, the next step should be percussion of the flanks. In order to detect flank dullness, approximately 1.5 L of fluid must be present. In fact, if there is no flank dullness, there is less than a 10% chance of having ascites. Once dullness of the flanks is appreciated, the clinician should then examine for shifting dullness that has 83% sensitivity for detecting ascites. It is important to note however the specificity is only approximately 50%.

Despite our knowledge of the clinical exam findings of ascites, physical exam maneuvers, by themselves, have only been shown to be accurate in about 50% of cases. In addition, physical examination results often have a high rate of false-positives and are especially problematic in obese patients. Thus, the diagnosis of ascites is often suspected on physical exam but should be confirmed on abdominal ultrasound.

The severity of ascites impacts its management. Mild ascites may only detectable by ultrasound. Moderate ascites could be considered when the ascites can be ascertained from the physical exam and causes symmetric distension of the abdomen, and severe is when the ascites is large or tense with marked abdominal distension.

Question 2. Once a diagnosis of ascites is made, how does one determine the cause of ascites? What is the differential diagnosis?

Ascites is fluid accumulation in the peritoneum. In the United States, the three most common causes of ascites are cirrhosis (85%), peritoneal malignancy (7%), and heart failure (3%). In addition, approximately 5% of patients have more than one cause of ascites.

The cause of ascites can be stratified using a diagnostic paracentesis. Per American Association for the Study of Liver Diseases (AASLD) and European Association for the Study of the Liver (EASL) guidelines, abdominal paracentesis should be performed in all new-onset ascites (both inpatient and outpatient).

The patient in this case underwent diagnostic paracentesis, and the fluid was sent for cell count and differential, albumin, and total protein. The results of our patient's diagnostic paracentesis are shown below:

Serum lab values:

- Albumin 2.7 g/dL
- Total protein 5.8 g/dL

Ascites lab values:

- Albumin 0.5 g/dL
- Total protein 1.5 g/dL

Once the decision has been made to perform a diagnostic paracentesis, the next decision is what labs to order. In uncomplicated ascites in which cirrhosis is suspected, only screening tests are necessary. These include a cell count and differential, albumin, and total protein. The gross appearance should also be noted (clear, purulent, bloody, chylous, etc.). If an ascitic fluid infection is suspected, the fluid should be cultured at bedside in aerobic and anaerobic blood culture bottles before initiating antibiotics. Of note, CA125 is not helpful in the differential diagnosis of ascites as it leads to unnecessary referrals and surgeries. The CA125 will be elevated in ascites as it is released from mesothelial cells when they are under pressure from the presence of ascitic fluid.

A serum-ascites albumin gradient (SAAG) and ascites protein levels are most useful for distinguishing among the three main causes of ascites (Table 3.1). A SAAG value of 1.1 or greater indicates that the ascites is due to portal hypertension (most common being either cirrhosis or heart failure). To calculate a SAAG, subtract the ascitic albumin concentration from the serum albumin concentration (should be collected on the same day). This simple calculation has 97% sensitivity and 90.2% specificity. In addition, an ascitic protein level of 2.5 g/dL or greater suggests heart failure as an etiology (53% sensitivity and 86.7% specificity). The difference in ascitic protein is due to the permeability of the hepatic sinusoids in both disease states. They are more permeable in heart failure-related ascites that allows protein-rich lymph to leak into the abdominal cavity.

Table 3.1 Diagnostic utility in serum-ascites albumin gradient and ascitic protein[a]

High albumin gradient (SAAG $\geq$1.1)		Low albumin gradient (SAAG <1.1)
Ascites protein <2.5 g/dL	Ascites protein >2.5 g/dL	
Cirrhosis Late Budd-Chiari	Heart failure Constrictive pericarditis Early Budd-Chiari	Malignancy Infectious Peritoneal tuberculosis Pancreatitis Nephrotic syndrome Protein-losing enteropathy

[a]Abbreviations: *SAAG* serum-ascites albumin gradient
Adapted from [10]

EASL guidelines also recommend using the ascitic protein level to help decide who will benefit from antibiotic prophylaxis from spontaneous bacterial peritonitis (SBP) as those with <1.5 g/dL of ascitic protein have an increased risk. Other indications for SBP prophylaxis include variceal hemorrhage and prior episode of SBP.

It is important to note also that those who have portal hypertension and a coexisting secondary cause of ascites formation (such as malignancy or tuberculosis) may also have a SAAG greater than or equal to 1.1. The SAAG also remains accurate despite either the administration of fluids or diuretics.

The results of his serum-ascites albumin gradient (SAAG) and ascitic total protein are consistent with a diagnosis of portal hypertension, most likely due to cirrhosis in this case.

Question 3: What is the management of ascites? What are the options once a patient fails to respond to initial medical management?

The first step in management of a patient with newly diagnosed ascites due to cirrhosis should be consideration of liver transplantation. At the first onset of ascites, the probability of survival is 85% during the first year but then drops to 56% at 5 years without a liver transplant. All patients should also be counseled on the importance of lifestyle changes and nutritional management. In fact, an evaluation by a nutritionist has been shown to reduce infection rates and perioperative mortality in cirrhotic patients. Alcohol abstinence in those with alcoholic liver disease is essential as it has drastic effects on prognosis and severity of ascites. For example, a clinical study which followed patients with Child-Pugh Class C alcoholic cirrhosis demonstrated that those who stopped alcohol use had their 3-year survival increase to 75%. In contrast, patient mortality was 100% at 3 years in those patients who continued to drink alcohol. In addition to the drastic mortality benefit, those who stop alcohol use may have ascites resolution or enhanced responsiveness to medical therapy.

An algorithm for the stepwise management of ascites is shown in Fig. 3.1. The first-line treatment for all detectable ascites is sodium restriction. The reason behind the importance of sodium restriction can be seen in the pathophysiology of ascites. In cirrhosis, portal hypertension causes splanchnic vasodilation that causes reduced effective arterial blood volume that triggers the kidneys to retain sodium causing fluid retention. Sodium restriction should be 2 gm or less a day. Although sodium restriction is

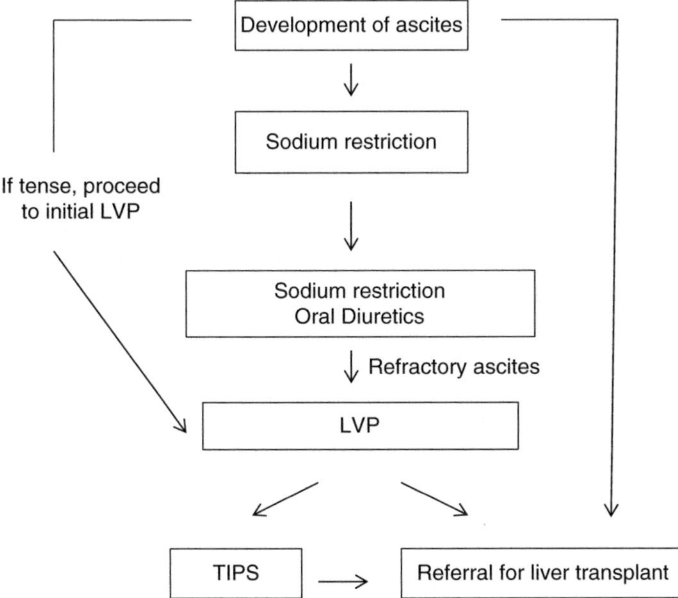

Fig. 3.1 Escalating management for ascites due to cirrhosis. (Abbreviations: LVP large volume paracentesis, TIPS transjugular intrahepatic portosystemic shunt)

essential, fluid restriction is not appropriate unless the patient has a hypervolemic hyponatremia with a serum sodium of <125 mEq/L.

Initiation of oral diuretics is effective in nearly 90% of patients with ascites without renal dysfunction. The recommended starting regimen is either spironolactone 100 mg alone or the combination of spironolactone and furosemide in a ratio of 100 mg to 40 mg (maintains normokalemia). Spironolactone selectively antagonizes the sodium-retaining effects of aldosterone and furosemide inhibits the Na/K/2Cl- cotransporter. The oral form of furosemide should always be used over intravenous (IV) due to the good oral bioavailability of furosemide and the fact that IV furosemide is associated with acute reductions in GFR in cirrhotic patients. The doses of spironolactone/furosemide can be titrated as an outpatient every 5–7 days based on weight loss (aiming for 0.5 kg of fluid loss per day once edema resolves), physical exam, renal function, and side effects. In addition, urine sodium can be used to assess the response; however, this is rarely done in the outpatient setting. The ratio of 100:40 should be maintained with dose titration with a maximum dose of 400 mg of spironolactone and 160 mg of furosemide. In terms of timing of dosing, a single morning dose maximizes compliance and decreases nocturia. Amiloride (10–40 mg per day) can be substituted for spironolactone in those with tender gynecomastia (however this medication has been shown to be less effective than spironolactone in a randomized controlled trial). Of note, hydrochlorothiazide should be avoided due to its ability to cause rapid development of hyponatremia. Furthermore, in moderate to severe ascites, it is reasonable to perform therapeutic paracentesis, followed by sodium restriction and oral diuretics.

Despite up-titration of diuretics and sodium restriction, refractory ascites can occur in nearly 10% of patients. Refractory ascites is defined as [18] ascites that is unresponsive to the highest intensity diuretic regimen (spironolactone 400 mg and furosemide 160 mg a day and a sodium-restricted diet) or [4] recurs rapidly after therapeutic paracentesis. Diuretic therapy is considered to have failed if there is minimal to no weight loss and no improvement in ascites or there are clinically significant diuretic-induced complications such as encephalopathy, serum creatinine >2 mg/dL, serum sodium <120 mEq/L, or serum potassium >6 mEq/L. In these cases, diuretics are usually stopped, and the patient is set up for large volume paracentesis (LVP). Patients will generally require paracentesis every 2–4 weeks (can be done as an outpatient). Per AASLD guidelines, if removing more than 5 L during a paracentesis, patients should receive additional volume expansion with intravenous (IV) albumin (6–8 gm per liter of ascites drained) in order to decrease the risk of circulatory dysfunction syndrome.

If a patient is requiring more than 2–3 LVPs in a month and does not respond to/tolerate maximum doses of diuretics, they should be evaluated for placement of a transjugular intrahepatic portosystemic shunt (TIPS). TIPS creates a low-resistance channel between the portal vein and hepatic vein which decreases portal pressure and, thus, ascites. There is growing evidence to consider TIPS in diuretic-resistant patients. Benefits include not only decreased ascitic volume but also decreased risk of SBP (by decreasing the need for LVPs) and a possible survival benefit. This is, however, offset somewhat by the risk of developing hepatic encephalopathy. Other treatment options include midodrine that has been shown to increase urine volume, urine sodium, MAP, and survival. It can be added to diuretics to increase blood pressure and help maintain a patient's sensitivity to diuretics.

The use of nonselective beta-blockers (NSBBs) in patients with ascites is controversial. There is concern about possible deleterious effects on the circulatory system and, subsequently, the renal system. To date, there hasn't been a randomized controlled trial, but observational studies do suggest that it is safe to use in those with ascites but that its dose should be carefully titrated. In the most recent 2016 AASLD guidelines, the society recommends avoiding doses of more than 160 mg of propranolol (or 80 mg of nadolol) when treating a patient with refractory ascites with careful monitoring for hypotension and its downstream effects. Additional studies are needed and clinical evaluation of its utility on a case-by-case basis is recommended.

Ascites itself can also lead to other potential complications in cirrhotic patients (Table 3.2). These include spontaneous bacterial peritonitis (discussed above), hepatic hydrothorax (due to the movement of ascetic fluid into the pleural space through defects in the diaphragm), umbilical hernias (due to the elevated abdominal pressure), and increased risk for intra-abdominal hypertension that is likely a mechanism in hepatorenal syndrome. Hepatic hydrothorax can occur in up to 4–12% of patients with cirrhosis and is classically a right-sided large transudative effusion. Management is often medical and includes sodium restriction, diuretics, and occasional therapeutic thoracentesis. Umbilical hernias can occur in up to 20% of cirrhotic patients and pose a surgical challenge as surgery can lead to wound infection, peritonitis, and wound dehiscence. Many studies have shown that treatment of ascites is essential in the treatment of the hernia and reduces complications if a surgical route is chosen. In terms of hepatorenal syndrome, elevated intra-abdominal pressures decreases renal blood flow, increases renal vascular resistance, and increases renal vein

Table 3.2 Complication of ascites

Abdominal discomfort (fullness after meals, decreased oral intake, dyspnea)
Spontaneous bacterial peritonitis
Umbilical hernia Inguinal hernia
Hepatic hydrothorax
Hepatorenal syndrome
Scrotal hydrocele
Post paracentesis complications (leak, hemorrhage)

pressures which decreases GFR and decreases urine output. Therefore, treatment of ascites has important clinical implications and decreases the risk of serious complications.

Conclusions

Ascites is the most common complication in patients with cirrhosis with approximately 60% of patients developing this fluid accumulation within 10 years of initial diagnosis of cirrhosis. With careful outpatient management, hospital admissions (and readmissions) can be reduced, and the care of these high-risk patients can be improved. The first step in management of ascites should always be consideration for liver transplantation due to its marker for high mortality. Management includes a comprehensive approach including lifestyle changes, titration of oral diuretics, and, if necessary, large volume paracentesis and TIPS.

Disclosure   The authors of this manuscript have no conflicts of interest to disclose.

Further Reading

1. Badillo R, Rockey DC. Hepatic hydrothorax. Medicine. 2014;93:135–42.
2. Biecker E. Diagnosis and therapy of ascites in liver cirrhosis. World J Gastroenterol. 2011;17(10):1237–48.
3. Boyer TD, Haskal ZJ. AASLD practice guidelines: the role of transjugular intrahepatic portosystemic shunt (TIPS) in the management of portal hypertension. Hepatology. 2010;51:1–16.
4. Cattau EL, Benjamin SB, Knuff TE, Castell DO. The accuracy of the physical examination in the diagnosis of suspected ascites. JAMA. 1982;247:1164–6.
5. Chang Y, Qi X, Li Z, Wang F, Wang S, Zhang Z, Xiao C, Ding T, Yang C. Int J Clin Exp Pathol. 2013;6:2523–8.

6. Coelho JCU, Claus CMP, Campos ACL, Costa MAR, Blum C. Umbilical hernia in patients with liver cirrhosis: a surgical challenge. World J Gastrointest Surg. 2016;8:476–82.

7. D-Amico G, Garcia-Tsao G, Pagliaro L. Natural history and prognostic indicators of survival in cirrhosis: a systematic review of 118 studies. J Hepatol. 2006;44:217–31.

8. Fortune B, Cardenas A. Ascites, refractory ascites and hyponatremia in cirrhosis. Gastroenterol Rep. 2017;5:104–12.

9. Garcia-Tsao G, Abraldes JG, Berzigotti A, Bosch J. Portal hypertensive bleeding in cirrhosis: risk stratification, diagnosis, and management: 2016 practice guidance by the American association for the study of liver diseases. Hepatology. 2017;65:310–35.

10. Hernaez R, Hamilton JP. Unexplained ascites. Am Assoc for the Study of Liver Dis. 2016;7:53–6.

11. Huang LL, Xia HHX, Zhu SL. Ascitic fluid analysis in the differential diagnosis of ascites: focus on cirrhotic ascites. J Clin Transl Hepatol. 2014;2:58–64.

12. EASL clinical practice guidelines: the management of ascites, spontaneous bacterial peritonitis, and hepatorenal syndrome in cirrhosis. J Hepatol. 2010;53:397–417.

13. Moctezuma-Velazquez C, Kalainy S, Abraldes JG. Beta-blockers in patients with advanced liver disease: has the dust settled? Liver Transpl. 2017;23:1058–69.

14. Patel YA, Muir AJ. Evaluation of new-onset ascites. JAMA. 2016;316:340–1.

15. Pose E, Cardenas A. Translating our current understanding of ascites management into new therapies for patients with cirrhosis and fluid retention. Dig Dis. 2017;35:402–10.

16. Runyon BA. AASLD practice guidelines: management of adult patients with ascites due to cirrhosis: update 2012. Am Assoc for the Study of Liver Dis. 2013;57:1651–3.

17. Runyon BA, Montano AA, Akriviadis EA, Antillon MR, Irving MA, McHutchison JG. The serum-ascites albumin gradient is superior to the exudate-transudate concept in the differential diagnosis of ascites. Ann Intern Med. 1992;117:215–20.

18. Williams JW, Simel DL. The rational clinical examination. Does this patient have ascites? How to divine fluid in the abdomen. JAMA. 1992;267:2645–8.

Chapter 4
Spontaneous Bacterial Peritonitis

Mona Hassan and Dilip Moonka

Introduction

Spontaneous bacterial peritonitis (SBP) is a common and potentially fatal infection of ascitic fluid in patients with cirrhosis. It is distinguished from secondary peritonitis by the absence of an evident intra-abdominal surgically treatable source. The prevalence of SBP is 10–30% in hospitalized patients with cirrhosis and ascites. Patients may present with symptoms such as abdominal pain, altered mental status, or fevers and chills. However, patients are often asymptomatic. In this chapter, we describe a case of SBP and discuss pathophysiology, diagnosis, treatment options, and outcomes.

Clinical Case Scenario

A 64-year-old male presents to the emergency department due to worsening abdominal distention and abdominal pain. He has a history of decompensated cirrhosis secondary to nonalcoholic fatty

M. Hassan
Department of Gastroenterology and Liver Disease, Henry Ford Hospital, Detroit, MI, USA

D. Moonka (✉)
Medical Director of Liver Transplantation, Division of Gastroenterology and Liver Disease, Henry Ford Hospital, Detroit, MI, USA
e-mail: dmoonka1@HFHS.org

© Springer Nature Switzerland AG 2019
S. M. Cohen, P. Davitkov (eds.), *Liver Disease*,
https://doi.org/10.1007/978-3-319-98506-0_4

liver disease (NAFLD) and is currently undergoing evaluation for liver transplantation. He denied any past surgical history. Review of systems was negative for fevers or chills and no changes in mental status. In addition, he denied any recent antibiotic use. His physical examination reveals scleral icterus and abdominal ascites. Labs revealed an ALT of 48 U/L (upper limit of normal of 35 U/L), AST of 66 U/L, bilirubin 2.5 mg/dL, albumin 2.8 g/dL, and INR 1.8. WBC was 10.4. Kidney function was within normal limits with a normal serum sodium level. A paracentesis was performed with the removal of 4 L of ascitic fluid. Ascites protein was 0.9 g/dL and ascites albumin was 0.4 g/dL. Fluid cell count revealed a WBC count of 623 with a polymorphonuclear (PMN) cell count of 61%.

Questions

1. What is the pathophysiology of SBP?
2. What are the potential risk factors for SBP?
3. How is SBP diagnosed?
4. What are the common organisms that cause in SBP?
5. What are the treatment options for this patient's SBP, and what are the expected cure rates and long-term prognosis?

Discussion

Question 1. What is the pathophysiology of SBP?

Patients with cirrhosis are predisposed to the development of bacterial overgrowth due to altered intestinal motility. In addition, cirrhosis may lead to increased intestinal permeability leading to bacterial translocation from the gut lumen and colonization of mesenteric lymph nodes. SBP can occur when the contaminated lymph nodes rupture due to high flow and high pressure due to portal hypertension. Alternatively, bacteria can translocate from mesenteric lymph nodes into the systemic circulation and then percolate through the liver into ascitic fluid. Cirrhosis itself is a form of acquired immune deficiency facilitating peritoneal infection.

Question 2. What are potential risk factors for SBP?

The majority of patients with SBP have advanced cirrhosis. In fact, the higher the model for end-stage liver disease (MELD) score, the greater the risk of SBP. Risk factors include any of the following: an ascitic fluid total protein concentration < 1 g/dL, serum total bilirubin >2.5 mg/dL, variceal bleeding, malnutrition, and a prior episode of SBP. The combination of certain features are also associated with an increased risk of SBP, which includes an ascitic fluid total protein <1.5 mg/dL with a Child-Pugh score $\geq$ 9 or with a serum creatinine of $\geq$1.2 mg/dL, BUN $\geq$25 mg/dL, or plasma sodium $\leq$130 mEq/L. Antibiotic prophylaxis should be considered for patients who meet these criteria. Options would include antibiotics such as Bactrim 1 double-strength tablet daily, norfloxacin 400 mg daily, or ciprofloxacin.

Question 3. How is SBP diagnosed?

Patients that present with abdominal pain or patients with ascites who are admitted to the hospital for other reasons should undergo paracentesis to look for evidence of SBP. A diagnostic paracentesis should not be delayed in patients with suspected SBP and should be performed, when possible, prior to the administration of antibiotic therapy. The diagnosis of SBP is based on the analysis of ascitic fluid. A diagnosis is made when the PMN cell count in the ascitic fluid is $\geq$250 cells/mm^3. Culture and gram

Table 4.1 Categories of SBP based on culture and cell count

Categories	Ascitic fluid culture	Absolute PMN/mm3
Spontaneous bacterial peritonitis	Positive	$\geq$250
Culture-negative neutrocytic ascites	No growth	$\geq$250
Monomicrobial non-neutrocytic bacterascites	Positive	<250
Polymicrobial bacterascites	Positive	<250

stain of the fluid should also be performed. The culture bottles should be inoculated at bedside to increase the yield.

Please refer to Table 4.1 regarding the classification of SBP and variants of SBP. In addition to classic SBP, there are three variants of SBP that are also "spontaneous" (there is no surgically treatable source for the infection): culture-negative neutrocytic ascites, monomicrobial non-neutrocytic bacterascites, and polymicrobial bacterascites. These variants are distinguished from classic SBP by ascitic fluid analysis.

1. SBP is characterized by a PMN count $\geq$250 and positive ascites cultures.
2. Culture-negative neutrocytic ascites has PMNs $\geq$250 but negative ascites cultures. This entity should be treated the same as SBP. It might reflect failure of prompt inoculation of the culture bottles at bedside. However, it is important to keep in mind that a number of other disorders can produce a somewhat similar picture including tuberculous peritonitis, malignancy-related ascites, and any process that attracts PMNs into the peritoneal cavity through the activation of cytokines such as tumor lysis syndrome.
3. Monomicrobial non-neutrocytic bacterascites occurs when the ascitic fluid PMN count is <250, but the ascites fluid culture is positive for one bacterial organism. This condition may progress to spontaneous bacterial peritonitis (SBP) or may resolve spontaneously in 62–86% of cases. Treatment

decisions for this entity depend on the clinical scenario. If symptomatic (fever or abdominal pain), they should be treated for infection. If asymptomatic, a repeat paracentesis could be considered in 48 h to assess for a rise in the ascitic PMN count.

4. Polymicrobial non-neutrocytic bacterascites occurs when the ascitic fluid PMN count is <250, but the ascites fluid culture is positive for multiple bacterial organisms. This variant is generally caused by a traumatic paracentesis in which bowel is entered by the paracentesis needle, and a (usually) transient bacterial leak occurs from the gut into the ascitic fluid. This complication can be recognized when air or frank stool is aspirated during attempted paracentesis or when multiple bacteria are identified on gram stain or on culture of non-neutrocytic ascites. This entity needs to be treated as an infection.

Question 4. What are the common organisms that cause SBP?

The three most common isolates in patients with SBP are *Escherichia coli*, *Klebsiella pneumoniae*, and *Streptococcus pneumoniae*. However, the widespread use of quinolones for prevention of SBP in high-risk groups, and frequent hospitalizations and exposure to broad-spectrum antibiotics, has led to changes in the organisms causing SBP with more gram-positive and extended-spectrum beta-lactamase-producing enterobacteriaceae. Risk factors for multi-resistant organisms include nosocomial infection, prolonged norfloxacin prophylaxis, recent infection, and recent antibiotic use.

Table 4.2 shows the data from one large study looking at the bacteria isolated in 519 SBP patients.

Table 4.2 Bacterial organisms isolated in patients with SBP in order of frequency

Organism	Percent of isolates
Escherichia coli	43
Klebsiella pneumoniae	11
Streptococcus pneumoniae	9
Other streptococcal species	19
Enterobacteriaceae	4
Staphylococcus	3
Pseudomonas	1
Miscellaneous	10

Question 5. What are the treatment options for this patient's SBP and, what are the expected cure rates and long-term prognosis?

Now that we have all of the baseline information and data on this patient, we can discuss treatment options. The best source for up-to-date information on SBP therapy is the AASLD guidelines. Broad-spectrum antibiotic therapy is recommended in patients with SBP until the susceptibility results are available. Third-generation cephalosporins such as ceftriaxone are recommended as initial therapy. In mild cases, oral therapy can be used and ofloxacin has been reported in a randomized controlled trial to be as effective as parenteral cefotaxime. Oral ciprofloxacin has also been found to be effective and more cost-effective than intravenous ceftazidime in a randomized trial. Therapy should be narrowed once susceptibilities are available.

Most would advocate repeating paracentesis at 48 h of therapy to confirm that the ascitic PMN count has decreased by >50%. If so, the treatment course can be stopped after 5 days of IV antibiotics.

Intravenous albumin should be administered in addition to antibiotic therapy. A landmark randomized-controlled trial revealed that patients who received cefotaxime plus 1.5 gm of albumin per kg body weight within 6 h of enrollment and 1.0 g/

kg on day 3 had a decrease in mortality from 29% to 10%. Recent data reveals that albumin should be given when the serum creatinine is >1 mg/dL, blood urea nitrogen >30 mg/dL, or total bilirubin >4 mg/dL but is not necessary in patients who do not meet these criteria.

Cure rates for SBP are very high, especially if the infection is diagnosed and treated early. However, if septic shock is present, in-hospital mortality can exceed 80%. Also, if there is renal dysfunction at the time of SBP diagnosis, the in-hospital mortality can approach 70%. Even in those who survive the initial bout of SBP, the long-term mortality is high. One- and 2-year mortality exceeds 50%. Thus, following a bout of SBP, patients should be considered for liver transplant options if they are reasonable candidates.

Although somewhat controversial, there may be increased mortality in patients who have SBP who remain on nonselective beta-blockers for portal hypertension complications. Permanently discontinuing the beta-blockers should be considered at the time of SBP diagnosis.

Based on the risk factors for SBP addressed in question # 2 above, our patient with a history of SBP should be placed on SBP prophylaxis once the active infection is treated.

Patient Treatment Course

The patient was treated with ceftriaxone 2 gm IV daily with improvement in his abdominal pain. Due to his low ascitic fluid total protein (less than 1.5 mg/dL) and Child-Pugh score of 10 and current SBP, he was subsequently placed on SBP prophylaxis with Bactrim 1 double-strength tablet daily. He was seen in hepatology clinic 3 weeks post discharge. He continues to have ascites, and therefore, his diuretic therapy was increased to spironolactone 100 mg daily and furosemide 40 mg daily. He has completed his transplant evaluation and is currently listed for transplant.

Conclusions

Spontaneous bacterial peritonitis is an infection of ascitic fluid in patients with cirrhosis. The prevalence is approximately 10–30% (including culture negative cases) in hospitalized patients with cirrhosis and ascites. Advanced liver disease, low ascitic protein, and previous SBP are risk factors. Enteric organisms such as *E. coli*, *Klebsiella pneumoniae*, and *Streptococcus pneumoniae* are the cause of SBP in 70% of cases. However, infection with resistant gram-positive extended-spectrum beta-lactamase bacteria can occur. A diagnostic paracentesis should be performed promptly in patients with suspected SBP. An ascitic fluid PMN count ≥ 250 is diagnostic of SBP. Once SBP is diagnosed, treatment with broad-spectrum antibiotics should be initiated immediately as mortality is decreased with early therapy. Prophylactic antibiotics are indicated after a bout of SBP to reduce recurrence. Patients who have had SBP should be considered for liver transplant options due to the high long-term mortality associated with this condition.

Further Reading

1. Ge PS, Runyon BA. Preventing future infections in cirrhosis: a battle cry for stewardship. Clin Gastroenterol Hepatol. 2015;13:760.
2. Guarner C, Runyon BA, Young S, Heck M, Sheikh MY. Translocation of gut bacteria in rats with cirrhosis to mesenteric lymph nodes partially explains the pathogenesis of spontaneous bacterial peritonitis. J Hepatol. 1997;26(6):1372.
3. http://www.aasld.org/practiceguidelines/Documents/ascitesupdate2013.pdf. Accessed 23 April 2013.
4. Kim JJ, Tsukamoto MM, Mathur AK, et al. Delayed paracentesis is associated with increased in-hospital mortality in patients with spontaneous bacterial peritonitis. Am J Gastroenterol. 2014;109:1436.

5. McHutchison JG, Runyon BA. Spontaneous bacterial peritonitis. In: Surawicz CM, Owen RL, editors. Gastrointestinal and hepatic infections. Philadelphia: WB Saunders; 1994. p. 455.
6. Runyon BA. Low-protein-concentration ascitic fluid is predisposed to spontaneous bacterial peritonitis. Gastroenterology. 1986;91(6):1343.
7. Runyon BA, AASLD. Introduction to the revised American Association for the Study of Liver Diseases practice guideline management of adult patients with ascites due to cirrhosis 2012. Hepatology. 2013;57:1651.
8. Runyon BA, Hoefs JC. Culture-negative neutrocytic ascites: a variant of spontaneous bacterial peritonitis. Hepatology. 1984;4:1209.
9. Runyon BA, Squier S, Borzio M. Translocation of gut bacteria in rats with cirrhosis to mesenteric lymph nodes partially explains the pathogenesis of spontaneous bacterial peritonitis. J Hepatol. 1994;21(5):792.
10. Salerno F, Navickis RJ, Wilkes MM. Albumin infusion improves outcomes of patients with spontaneous bacterial peritonitis: a meta-analysis of randomized trials. Clin Gastroenterol Hepatol. 2013;11:123.
11. Sigal SH, Stanca CM, Fernandez J, Arroyo V, Navasa M. Restricted use of albumin for spontaneous bacterial peritonitis. Gut. 2007;56(4):597–9.

Chapter 5
Hepatorenal Syndrome

Yumi Ando and Joseph Ahn

Introduction

Renal failure is a common cause of death in patients with end-stage liver disease. The key distinguishing feature of the hepatorenal syndrome (HRS) is its occurrence in the setting of portal hypertension and subsequent ascites formation. After the onset of ascites, the probability of developing HRS is 18% at 1 year and 39% at 5 years. For the hospitalized patient with cirrhosis and ascites, 20% develop some form of acute kidney injury (AKI). Twenty percent of those patients have HRS. The prognosis of untreated HRS is abysmally poor and spontaneous recovery is unlikely. If untreated, the expected survival for type I HRS is 2 weeks and 6 months for type II HRS. This chapter will enable clinicians to recognize patients at risk for developing HRS, rapidly diagnose the condition by excluding other etiologies of AKI, and initiate treatment promptly to improve clinical outcomes.

Y. Ando (✉) · J. Ahn
Department of Medicine, Division of Gastroenterology and Hepatology,
Oregon Health and Science University, Portland, OR, USA
e-mail: andoy@ohsu.edu

© Springer Nature Switzerland AG 2019
S. M. Cohen, P. Davitkov (eds.), *Liver Disease*,
https://doi.org/10.1007/978-3-319-98506-0_5

Y. Ando and J. Ahn

Clinical Case Scenario

A 58-year-old man with cirrhosis due to nonalcoholic steatohepatitis presents to the emergency room. He was urged by his PCP to go to the hospital after routine labs demonstrated an increase in his serum creatinine from a baseline value of 0.8 mg/dL to 3.0 mg/dL. He is otherwise asymptomatic. He has large ascites requiring weekly large-volume paracenteses (LVP). His last LVP was 3 days ago and 6 L of ascites was removed with appropriate IV albumin replacement. Ascitic cell count and culture from this sample were negative for spontaneous bacterial peritonitis. He is currently not on diuretics to treat ascites due to chronic hyponatremia with a recent serum Na of 125 mEq/L. He denies taking any nonsteroidal anti-inflammatory drugs. He also denies drinking alcohol or using herbal or dietary supplements. The only medication he currently takes is lactulose. He has been having three formed brown stools daily and has had good oral intake.

Upon arrival to the emergency room, his vital signs were temperature of 98.3 F, pulse 70, respirations 18, and blood pressure of 89/45 mmHg (mean arterial pressure of 60 mmHg). None of his vital signs were particularly off from his baseline values. On examination, he has slight scleral icterus, gynecomastia, large but not tense ascites, palmar erythema, and numerous spider angiomata on his face and chest. Urinalysis demonstrates a bland urine sediment with no white blood cells, red blood cells, casts, or protein. He is given 100 g of IV albumin and is admitted to the medicine service. The next day, his serum Cr has increased again to 4.5 mg/dL.

Clinical Questions

1. What is the differential diagnosis of a patient with cirrhosis presenting with acute kidney injury?
2. How is HRS diagnosed? What work-up should be initiated when HRS is suspected?
3. What causes HRS?

4. Can HRS be prevented?
5. What is the best treatment strategy for HRS?
6. If medical treatment for HRS fails, what next?

Discussion

Question 1. What is the differential diagnosis of a patient with cirrhosis presenting with acute kidney injury?

Kidney injury can occur due to a variety of insults in the cirrhotic patient. Kidney injury can largely be divided into prerenal, intrinsic renal, and postrenal etiologies. Commonly encountered etiologies in cirrhotic patients are summarized in Table 5.1.

Table 5.1 Common etiologies for acute kidney injury in patients with cirrhosis

Etiology	Classification	Comments
Hepatorenal syndrome	Prerenal	Decreased renal perfusion due to increased renal vascular tone and low effective circulating volume
Hypovolemia	Prerenal	GI hemorrhage, diarrhea from excessive lactulose, poor PO intake due to hepatic encephalopathy
Acute tubular necrosis	Intrinsic renal	Sustained hypotension due to sepsis, aminoglycosides. Muddy brown granular casts can be seen in urinalysis, though not always
Membranoproliferative glomerulonephritis	Intrinsic renal	Seen in patients with chronic HCV and HBV. Urinalysis with dysmorphic red cells and red cell casts
Diabetic nephropathy	Intrinsic renal	Seen commonly in patients with nonalcoholic steatohepatitis with concomitant diabetes. Albuminuria
Obstructive nephropathy	Postrenal	Obstruction can occur anywhere along the urinary tract. Commonly seen in older men with prostatic hypertrophy or carcinoma

When diagnosing AKI in cirrhotic patients, keep in mind that even a small increase in serum creatinine (SCr) can correlate with a significant decrease in glomerular filtration rate (GFR). SCr may overestimate a cirrhotic patient's GFR due to the sarcopenia that often occurs in the setting of severe protein calorie malnutrition in end-stage liver disease. In 2015, the International Ascites Club revised the definition of AKI in cirrhosis as an increase in SCr of 0.3 mg/dL within 48 h or a 50% increase or more in SCr from a baseline within 3 months.

Question 2. How is HRS diagnosed? What work-up should be initiated when HRS is suspected?

HRS is diagnosed if all criteria are met in Table 5.2. Because there are no well-defined biomarkers that can establish the diagnosis of HRS, it is a diagnosis of exclusion. Thus, it is crucial to take a detailed history to investigate the possibility of other etiologies of kidney injury. The history should include exposure to nephrotoxic agents. Commonly seen nephrotoxic agents include

Table 5.2 Diagnostic criteria for hepatorenal syndrome

Cirrhosis with ascites
Serum creatinine >1.5 mg/dL
Absence of shock: note that patients can have an active infection as long as it is not causing distributive shock
Absence of hypovolemia as defined by lack of sustained improvement of renal function following at least 48 h of diuretic withdrawal and volume expansion with albumin 1 g/kg/day up to a maximum of 100 g/day
No current or recent treatment with nephrotoxic agents
Absence of parenchymal renal disease as defined by proteinuria <0.5 g/day, microhematuria <50 RBC/HPF, and normal renal ultrasound

NSAIDS, antibiotics, and IV radiocontrast. Much can be assessed regarding a patient's volume status by asking about fluid losses from excessive diuresis, diarrhea, vomiting, poor oral intake, or GI blood loss. Infectious symptoms should also be asked as part of the review of systems. Physical exam should focus on evidence of ascites and estimation of volume status. Urine output should be closely monitored – insertion of a Foley catheter may be necessary if the patient is unable to cooperate with urine collection. Laboratory work-up should include CBC, CMP, INR, urinalysis with microscopic examination of the urinary sediment, and spot urine sodium and creatinine to calculate the fractional excretion of sodium (FENa). If the patient was recently exposed to diuretics, spot urine urea should also be obtained to calculate the fractional excretion of urea (FEUrea). Infectious work-up including ascites cell count and culture, even in asymptomatic patients, should be performed. In cases when obstructive uropathy is suspected, a renal ultrasound should also be performed.

Two types of hepatorenal syndrome have been described based on the rapidity of the decline in kidney function. However, it is unclear if there is any difference in the underlying pathophysiology.

Type I HRS
- At least a twofold increase in serum creatinine to a level greater than 2.5 mg/dL (221 micromol/L) over a period of <2 weeks without sustained improvement in renal function (<20% decrease in Cr) at least 48 h after diuretic withdrawal and albumin fluid challenge

Type II HRS
- Slow progression of renal function impairment with avid sodium retention and refractory ascites. Can transition to type I HRS at any time with or without an identifiable trigger

Question 3. What causes HRS?

Cirrhosis leads to increased intrahepatic vascular resistance and subsequent portal hypertension. This triggers an increase in splanchnic production of vasodilators such as nitric oxide. This splanchnic arterial vasodilation decreases effective circulating blood volume and arterial blood pressure. It also causes ascites by increasing the splanchnic capillary hydrostatic pressure leading to splanchnic lymph formation that exceeds lymph return. Decreased circulating blood volume causes activation of the sympathetic nervous system, vasopressin, and the renin-angiotensin-aldosterone system (RAAS). This leads to sodium and water retention causing increased plasma volume, impaired free water excretion causing dilutional hyponatremia, and renal vasoconstriction. Hepatorenal syndrome occurs when the compensatory mechanisms fail to maintain appropriate cardiac output despite maximal renal vasoconstriction, leading to poor renal vascular blood flow and decreased glomerular filtration rate.

Question 4. Can HRS be prevented?

There is currently no prophylactic therapy for the prevention of HRS, although measures can be taken to prevent common precipitating events. The most common precipitators of HRS are:

- Bacterial infection (especially SBP)
- Gastrointestinal bleeding
- Acute alcoholic hepatitis
- LVP without appropriate albumin replacement

It is crucial to recognize these events and take appropriate measures so that they can be treated rapidly before renal dysfunction occurs.

Spontaneous bacterial peritonitis is the most common bacterial infection precipitating HRS. The appropriate treatment of

SBP and secondary prophylaxis will be discussed elsewhere in this book and will not be covered in this chapter. As HRS occurs in 30% of patients who develop SBP, primary antibiotic prophylaxis is recommended in patients who are at particular risk of developing HRS. Several studies have demonstrated that patients with low ascites protein (<1.5 g/L) with Child-Turcotte-Pugh (CTP) score $\geq$ 9 and bilirubin $\geq$3 or impaired renal function (SCr $\geq$ 1.2 mg/dL, BUN $\geq$25 mg/dL, or serum Na $\leq$ 130 mEq/L) who receive norfloxacin antibiotic prophylaxis have significantly decreased mortality as well as a 1-year probability of developing SBP or HRS. In a similar vein, GI hemorrhage often leads to infectious complications in patients with cirrhosis which can then lead to HRS. Prophylactic antibiotics used for 7 days for patients with cirrhosis who suffer GI hemorrhage have been shown to decrease infectious complications by 30% and improve overall survival.

Ideally, alcoholic hepatitis is prevented by adequate community resources and support to achieve patient sobriety. However, if it does occur, recognition of the severity followed by rapid treatment with prednisolone as indicated, nutritional support, and fluid management can sometimes prevent the onset of HRS.

When removing more than 5 L of ascites with a LVP, 6–8 g of IV albumin per liter of fluid removed has demonstrated decrease in post-paracentesis circulatory dysfunction (defined as an increase in plasma renin activity of 50% or greater). This may prevent HRS, as well as decrease overall mortality.

Question 5. What is the best treatment strategy for HRS?

The mainstay of HRS therapy is vasoactive agents combined with colloid volume expansion with albumin. A list of medications that are used for HRS is described in Table 5.3. Answering the question of which treatment strategy is superior is difficult

Table 5.3 Medical therapy for the treatment of hepatorenal syndrome: goal of therapy is sustained decrease in serum Cr to <1.5 mg/dL

Treatment	Definition	Dosing
Terlipressin	Analogue of vasopressin (ADH) that acts on V1 vasopressin receptor and increases SVR. It has relative specificity for the splanchnic circulation, thus reducing portal HTN	0.5–2 mg IV bolus every 4–6 h, titrate until MAP increases by $\geq$ 10 mmHg or MAP $\geq$ 80 mmHg
Norepinephrine	Alpha-1- and beta-1-adrenergic agonist causing increased cardiac contractility, heart rate, and systemic vasoconstriction. The alpha effects (vasoconstriction)> > beta effects (inotropy and chronotropy)	0.5–3 mg/hr given as a continuous IV infusion, titrate until MAP increases by $\geq$ 10 mmHg or MAP $\geq$ 80 mmHg
Midodrine	Alpha-1-adrenergic agonist causing systemic as well as splanchnic vasoconstriction by increasing vascular tone	7.5–15 mg PO TID, titrate until MAP increases by $\geq$ 10 mmHg or MAP $\geq$ 80 mmHg
Octreotide	Somatostatin analogue that inhibits the secretion of glucagon and enhances splanchnic vasoconstriction by inhibiting glucagon-mediated splanchnic vasodilation	100–200 mcg SQ TID or 50 mcg/hr continuous IV infusion

due to the lack of high-quality evidence. Terlipressin has been the most extensively studied, and a number of randomized placebo controlled double-blinded trials have been reported. However, many had small study populations despite being multicenter trials because of difficulty in identifying and enrolling HRS patients. Some studies showed resolution of HRS or at least some improvement in renal function, although all were not powered to demonstrate a survival benefit. A Cochrane systematic review of terlipressin vs. placebo combining data from five randomized controlled trials did show a survival benefit of terlipressin compared to controls. It is important to keep in mind that terlipressin is currently not commercially available in the United States because it has not been approved by the US Food and Drug Administration. The drug is currently awaiting the results of a phase 3 "CONFIRM" clinical trial to assess the safety and efficacy of the drug. The study should be completed in 2019.

In countries where terlipressin is not available, the treatment options include norepinephrine or a combination of midodrine and octreotide. Administration of norepinephrine requires intensive care monitoring due to the need for close titration of the drug and risk of cardiovascular and ischemic complications. On the other hand, midodrine and octreotide can be given on a regular hospital ward. They can even be safely administered at home as midodrine is given orally and octreotide can be given subcutaneously. A head-to-head comparison trial between terlipressin and midodrine + octreotide in Italy was terminated early after interim analysis showed a significantly higher rate of renal recovery in the terlipressin group. Several trials comparing terlipressin to norepinephrine showed no difference in HRS reversal. Although more high-quality studies are needed, current evidence points toward norepinephrine as being the treatment of choice in cases where terlipressin is not available.

Question 6. If medical treatment for HRS fails, what next?

Even with maximal medical support, HRS reversal only occurs in 40–50% of patients. In addition, HRS reversal with medical therapy has shown improvement in short-term mortality in some studies, but there is no evidence of improvement in long-term survival. At present, the only treatment that provides long-term survival for patients with HRS is liver transplantation. Consequently, pharmacologic therapy and renal replacement therapy are seen as a bridge to transplantation. A recent retrospective cohort study found that patients with HRS who were not listed for liver transplant had an 85% mortality despite initiation of renal replacement therapy (RRT). Although the decision to initiate RRT in patients with HRS not approved for liver transplantation who are unresponsive to medical therapy is nuanced and can be considered in certain cases, in general, the risk of RRT outweighs the benefit and is not offered. In such cases, best supportive care and palliation are recommended.

Transjugular intrahepatic portosystemic shunt (TIPS) has been shown to reverse HRS in small pilot studies and can be considered in situations where no other options exist and as a bridge to liver transplantation. However, we must keep in mind that the patients included in these studies were a highly selected group due to strict exclusion criteria (INR > 2, Bili >5 mg/dL, CTP score > 12, portal vein thrombosis, and active infection within the last 2 weeks). In reality, most patients who develop HRS would not meet this criteria. In addition, given the risk of hepatic encephalopathy and further liver decompensation due to hepatic ischemia, especially in patients with MELD score > 18, the decision to proceed with TIPS should be weighed carefully.

Patients with type I HRS who undergo liver transplantation often have significant improvement in renal function within several months of transplant. For the most part, patients who required RRT pretransplant will not require long-term dialysis posttransplant. For those with type II HRS, simultaneous liver-kidney (SLK) transplantation can be considered due to the concern that these patients may have developed irreversible kidney injury requiring posttransplant long-term dialysis. However, offering SLK transplant for HRS is highly controversial. Furthermore, it is unknown if there is a survival benefit to offering SLK vs. liver transplant (LT) alone in patients with HRS. Rates of SLK differ significantly between transplant centers due to the lack of studies comparing their safety and efficacy compared to LT alone. In an effort to standardize the use of SLK, the United Network for Organ Sharing (UNOS) has recently established a set of eligibility criteria for SLK transplant allocation as follows:

- CKD with GFR $\leq$ 60 ml/min for >90 consecutive days and on regular dialysis or GFR < 35 ml/min at time of listing
- Sustained AKI defined as dialysis dependent for at least 6 consecutive weeks or GFR < 25 ml/min for 6 consecutive weeks
- Metabolic disease of one of the following: hyperoxaluria, atypical HUS, familial non-neuropathic systemic amyloid, and methylmalonic aciduria

There is also a "safety net" for those who do not meet the above criteria but have significant renal dysfunction. During 2–12 months after liver transplantation, if the patient's GFR remains $\leq$20 ml/min or remains dependent on dialysis, they will obtain priority for kidney transplantation above patients listed for only kidney transplants.

Patient's Clinical Course

This patient's work-up revealed a urine Na of 4 mmol/L and FENa of <1%. Renal ultrasound did not demonstrate obstruction of the urinary tract. Pan-infectious work-up including blood, urine, and ascites culture was negative. Despite volume expansion with IV albumin for 48 h, there was no improvement in serum Cr. His urine sediment continued to be bland. He was started on midodrine, octreotide, and albumin as terlipressin was not available for routine use in the United States. However, his serum creatinine continued to rise and his urine output decreased to <500 ml/day. He was transferred to the intensive care unit where norepinephrine infusion was started and titrated to increase mean arterial pressure by 10 mmHg. His serum Cr decreased slowly but continued to be >1.5 mg/dL. At the same time, urgent inpatient liver transplant evaluation was initiated by the hepatology team. His case was discussed at selection conference where no contraindications were identified and he was deemed a good transplant candidate. His MELD-Na at the time of listing was 35. Five days after being placed on the waiting list, an acceptable organ offer became available and the patient underwent successful orthotopic liver transplantation. Six weeks after transplantation, he was seen in the hepatology clinic where serum Cr was noted to be 1.3 mg/dL.

Conclusions

Renal dysfunction, regardless of etiology, is a strong independent risk factor for mortality in patients with end-stage liver disease. This is reflected in the degree of weight the serum creatinine carries in the MELD allocation score. Studies have also demonstrated that pretransplant renal dysfunction leads to worse post-transplant survival, especially in those who required pretransplant RRT. Early recognition of HRS is crucial so that treatment can be initiated rapidly in the hopes of avoiding RRT. Even when appropriately recognized and treated, the 3-month survival with type I and II HRS is 20% and 40%, respectively. Thus, patients diagnosed with HRS should undergo or be referred for liver transplant evaluation expeditiously. We hope that this chapter will provide the tools needed to diagnose HRS in a timely manner so that more patients can undergo liver transplantation, rather than dying before they can be considered for transplant evaluation.

Further Reading

1. AASLD Practice guideline: management of adult patients with ascites due to cirrhosis: Update 2012.
2. Allegretti AS, et al. Prognosis of patients with cirrhosis and AKI who initiate RRT. Clin J Am Soc Nephrol. 2018;13(1):16–25.
3. Gines A, et al. Incidence, predictive factors, and prognosis of the hepatorenal syndrome in cirrhosis with ascites. Gastroenterology. 1993;105(1):229–36.

4. Gluud L, et al. Terlipressin for hepatorenal syndrome. Cochrane Database Syst Rev. 2012;12(9):CD005162.
5. Israelsen M, et al. Terlipressin vs other vasoactive drugs for hepatorenal syndrome. Cochrane Database Syst Rev Issue. 2017;27(9):CD011532.
6. EASL practice guideline: EASL clinical practice guidelines on the management of ascites, spontaneous bacterial peritonitis, and hepatorenal syndrome in cirrhosis. J Hepatol. 53:397–417.
7. Modi RM, et al. Outcomes of liver transplantation in patients with hepatorenal syndrome. World J Hepatol. 2016;8(24):999–1011.
8. Nazar A, et al. Predictors of response to therapy with terlipressin and albumin in patients with cirrhosis and type 1 hepatorenal syndrome. Hepatology. 2010;51(1):219–26.
9. Salermo F, et al. Diagnosis, prevention, and treatment of hepatorenal syndrome in cirrhosis. Gut. 2007;56(9):1310–8.
10. Wong F, et al. Working party proposal for a revised classification system of renal dysfunction in patients with cirrhosis. Gut. 2011;60(5):702–9.

Chapter 6
Chronic Hepatitis B

Lindsay Meurer and Anthony Post

Introduction

Hepatitis B (HBV) is a viral infection of the liver and a common cause of chronic liver disease worldwide. An estimated 240 million people are affected by chronic hepatitis B (CHB) infection globally. In the United States, 850,000 to 2.2 million are estimated to be living with HBV. Screening and vaccination efforts have been globally implemented to reduce the burden of disease. This chapter will focus on the diagnosis and management of CHB.

L. Meurer
University Hospitals Cleveland Medical, Center Case Western
Reserve University, Cleveland, OH, USA
e-mail: Lindsay.Meurer@UHhospitals.org

A. Post
Division of Gastroenterology and Liver Disease, University Hospitals
Cleveland Medical Center, Case Western Reserve University,
Cleveland, OH, USA

© Springer Nature Switzerland AG 2019   61
S. M. Cohen, P. Davitkov (eds.), *Liver Disease*,
https://doi.org/10.1007/978-3-319-98506-0_6

Clinical Case Scenario

A 39-year-old woman presents to her primary care practitioner's office for evaluation of right upper quadrant discomfort after eating fried foods. She was born in Hong Kong and moved to the United States with her parents in 1985. She is an elementary school teacher. She has never used intravenous drugs and rarely consumes alcohol. She has had three lifetime sexual partners but has been monogamous with her husband since they got married 10 years ago. She has two children who are in good health. She takes no medications. There is no family history of hepatocellular carcinoma (HCC). On exam, she is healthy appearing without right upper quadrant tenderness, ascites, or peripheral edema. An ultrasound of the liver reveals gallstones in the gallbladder and a normal appearing liver. Her liver function panel reveals AST 120 U/L, ALT 179 U/L, alkaline phosphatase 120 U/L, and total bilirubin 0.6 mg/dL. Her viral hepatitis panel reveals hepatitis B surface antigen (HBsAg) positive, hepatitis B surface antibody (HBsAb) negative, hepatitis B core IgM negative, and hepatitis C antibody negative. She is referred to a liver specialist for further evaluation and management of her HBV.

Questions

1. How do you approach a patient found to be HBsAg positive? What other testing is indicated at this time? How will you interpret the results of testing?
2. With regard to disease transmission, what advice should you give this patient?
3. What are the treatment recommendations for patients with HBV?
4. What is the recommended follow-up for patients with CHB? Should CHB patients be screened for HCC?

Discussion

Question 1. How do you approach a patient found to be HBsAg positive? What other testing is indicated at this time? How will you interpret the results of testing?

Correct interpretation of hepatitis B serologic testing is important in determining chronicity of infection and disease susceptibility. HBsAg is the main serologic marker of HBV infection. The development of antibodies to HBsAg signifies disease recovery or previous vaccination. Hepatitis B e antigen (HBeAg) is an indicator of infectivity and active viral replication. Hepatitis B core antibody (anti-HBc) develops early in HBV infection (as HBcIgM) and remains present lifelong (as HBcIgG or HBc total antibody). See Table 6.1 below for summary of HBV serology interpretation.

Table 6.1 Interpretation of HBV serologic testing

Test	Result	Interpretation
HBsAg Anti-HBc Anti-HBs	Negative Negative Negative	Negative (not infected or vaccinated)
HBSAg Anti-HBc Anti-HBs	Negative **Positive** **Positive**	Resolved HBV infection
HBSAg Anti-HBc Anti-HBs	Negative Negative **Positive**	Vaccinated
HBSAg Anti-HBc Anti-HBs	**Positive** **Positive** Negative	Active HBV infection (usually chronic) If anti-HBc IgM present, may represent acute infection
HBSAg Anti-HBc Anti-HBs	Negative **Positive** Negative	1. Distant resolved infection (most common) 2. Recovering acute infection 3. False positive 4. Occult "low-level" CHB

Our patient presents with biliary colic but is incidentally found to have elevated transaminases and a positive HBsAg. CHB infection is defined as HBsAg positivity for greater than 6 months. Most people with CHB are asymptomatic without evidence of liver disease at the time of diagnosis. Initial evaluation should include a focused history and physical examination aiming to identify signs or symptoms of cirrhosis, alcohol use or other metabolic risk factors for liver disease, personal or family history of HBV or HCC, and potential risk factors for disease acquisition.

Initial laboratory evaluation should include CBC, liver function studies (AST, ALT, bilirubin, alkaline phosphatase, albumin), and PT/INR. Additional serologic testing should include hepatitis B e antigen (HBeAg), anti-HBe antibody, and HBV DNA quantification. Unlike hepatitis C, HBV genotype testing is not necessary at initial evaluation. Antibodies to hepatitis A, D (delta), and C should also be measured in order to exclude coinfection and determine the need for vaccination against HAV. HIV screening is essential because of the similar transmission patterns with HBV. Current antiviral regimens against HBV also have activity against HIV which may lead to the development of resistance strains of HIV if only treated with a single agent. A liver ultrasound should be routinely performed to evaluate the liver parenchyma and screen for liver cancer. An alpha-fetoprotein (AFP) level can also be measured as part of HCC surveillance.

The degree of liver fibrosis can also be assessed in order to provide risk stratification of disease progression and assist with management decisions. However, the various CHB treatment guidelines differ on the need for liver biopsy before deciding on therapy. Liver biopsy is regarded as the best method to assess liver histology; however, in many cases, noninvasive strategies can be used. For example, serum markers of fibrosis include AST-to-platelet ratio index (APRI), FIB-4, and FibroTest©. Additionally, the ultrasound-based modality of vibration-controlled transient elastography (FibroScan©) can be used to assess liver fibrosis. These noninvasive measures are useful in excluding advanced fibrosis but only have moderate accuracy in detecting lesser degrees of fibrosis. Liver biopsy is often performed to determine the degree of fibrosis and inflammation if this information is not readily apparent from the initial blood work or results are discordant with the clinical picture of disease.

Our patient in the clinical case scenario underwent appropriate initial testing with results as follows:

CBC: Within normal limits, including a normal platelet count
PT: Normal, INR 1.0
Albumin: 3.8 g/dL
Hepatitis e antigen: Positive
Hepatitis e antibody: Nonreactive
Hepatitis B DNA: 50,000 IU/mL
Hepatitis A total antibody: Nonreactive
Hepatitis D antibody: Nonreactive
HIV: Negative
AFP: 4 ng/mL
APRI index: no fibrosis
FibroScan: stage 1–2 fibrosis

With the above information, we can classify our patient into one of the four phases of CHB infection as outlined in Table 6.2 as taken from the American Association for the Study of Liver Disease (AASLD) Guidelines for the treatment of CHB.

Our patient's initial serologic testing is consistent with CHB infection given the presence of HBsAg and negative core IgM antibody. As discussed earlier, to be classified as CHB the HBsAg should be present for at least 6 months, however in patients born in endemic regions, a single positive HBsAg is considered indicative of CHB. Our patient is also HBeAg positive with a high HBV viral load and an elevated ALT, which classifies her infection as being in the immune active phase. She does not have any stigmata of cirrhosis on examination and no

Table 6.2 Phases of CHB infection

Phase	ALT	HBV DNA	HBeAg	Liver histology
Immune tolerant	Normal[a]	Elevated, >1 million IU/mL	Positive	Minimal inflammation and fibrosis
HBeAg positive, immune active	Elevated	Elevated, ≥20,000 IU/mL	Positive	Moderate-severe inflammation or fibrosis
Inactive CHB	Normal	Low or undetectable, <2000 IU/mL	Negative	Minimal necroinflammation, variable fibrosis
HBeAg-negative, immune reactivation	Elevated	Elevated, ≥2000 IU/mL	Negative	Moderate-severe inflammation or fibrosis

[a]It is important to note that for the purposes of CHB evaluation, the AASLD defines normal values of ALT as <19 U/L for females and < 30 U/L for males

laboratory evidence of decreased liver synthetic function or portal hypertension. Noninvasive measure confirms mild-moderate fibrosis without evidence of cirrhosis; therefore liver biopsy is not indicated.

Question 2. With regard to disease transmission, what advice should you give this patient?

HBV can be transmitted perinatally or through activities involving percutaneous or mucosal contact with infectious blood or body fluids. The most common mode of transmission in endemic areas such as Asia, sub-Saharan Africa, or Alaska is through vertical transmission from infected mother to child. Common modes of transmission in non-endemic countries such as the United States include sexual intercourse with infected partner, injection drug use involving shared needles or syringes, direct close contact with blood or open sores of an infected person, and needle sticks or sharp instrument exposure. HBV is not spread through food or water, sharing eating utensils, kissing, or coughing. The likelihood of developing CHB depends largely on an individual's age of acquisition. When transmitted vertically, 90% of infected infants will proceed to develop CHB. In contrast, only 2–6% of those who acquire the disease in adulthood will develop CHB.

Our patient's risk factors for HBV acquisition include birth in an endemic region and possible sexual transmission. To reduce the risk of transmitting infection to household contacts, our patient should be advised to avoid sharing razors and toothbrushes. Blood should be treated as infectious and cleaned using gloves and bleach-containing solution. Sexual partners and children should be referred for hepatitis B screening including HBsAg, anti-HBs, and anti-HBc. If not immune, vaccines should be given.

Other groups that benefit from HBV screening are listed in Table 6.3. Vaccination is recommended universally during infancy and is especially important in the high-risk populations listed below.

Table 6.3 Persons who should be screened for HBV

Persons born in countries with 2% or higher HBV prevalence (Asia, sub-Saharan Africa, Alaska, northern providences of Canada, and Greenland)
Men who have sex with men
Injection drug users
HIV-infected persons
Household and sexual contacts of HBV-infected persons
Persons requiring immunosuppressive therapy
Persons with end-stage renal disease
Blood and tissue donors
Persons infected with hepatitis C
Persons with elevated transaminases
Incarcerated persons
Pregnant women
Infants born to HBV-infected mothers

Questions 3. What are the treatment recommendations for patients with CHB?

Among untreated adults with HBV, 8–20% go on to develop cirrhosis. Among those with cirrhosis, the 5-year risk of decompensated liver disease is 20% and risk of developing HCC is 2–5%. The goal of therapy for CHB is reducing morbidity and mortality through prevention of liver disease progression. HBV cannot be totally eliminated or cured because HBV DNA is integrated into the host genome. Surrogate markers signify treatment response and viral suppression. An immunologic response is defined as sustained reduction in HBV DNA to undetectable levels with the ultimate goal being loss of HBsAg and acquisition of surface antibody. Unfortunately, loss of HBsAg is rarely achieved with current treatment options. Biochemical and histologic response involve normalization of ALT and decrease in liver inflammation and fibrosis. The decision to treat is complex and considers many variables including the phase of CHB, presence or absence of cirrhosis, and risk of disease progression.

Table 6.4 outlines the indications for CHB treatment according to the European Association for the Study of Liver Disease (EASL) and AASLD clinical practice guidelines.

There are two primary CHB treatment options currently available: nucleotide/side analogues (NA) or pegylated interferon-alpha (PEG-IFNα). When compared directly, a single antiviral agent has not shown superiority in reducing liver-related complications of CHB. Decisions in treatment must be individualized and take into account comorbid conditions, renal function, desire for finite therapy, family planning, and medication cost. The AASLD recommends PEG-IFNα, entecavir, or tenofovir as preferred initial treatment in adults with CHB based upon reduced risk of developing resistance during treatment. Combination therapy is not recommended. The main advantages of NA therapy include an oral route of administration, predictable viral

Table 6.4 Indications for treatment of CHB

Patient characteristics	AASLD (2016)	EASL (2017)
HBeAg positive	HBV DNA >20,000 IU/mL, ALT >2x ULN	HBV DNA >2000 IU/mL, ALT >ULN, and/or at least moderate liver necroinflammation or fibrosis
HBeAg negative	HBV DNA >2000 IU/mL, ALT >2x ULN	HBV DNA >2000 IU/mL, ALT >ULN, and/or at least moderate liver necroinflammation or fibrosis
Compensated cirrhosis	HBV DNA >2000 IU/mL regardless of ALT levels	Any detectable HBV DNA regardless of ALT levels
Decompensated cirrhosis	All patients	Any detectable HBV DNA regardless of ALT levels
Other	Adults >40, normal ALT, HBV DNA $\geq$ 1,000,000 IU/mL with significant necroinflammation or fibrosis	Patients with HBV DNA >20,000 IU/mL and ALT >2x ULN regardless of degree of fibrosis

suppression, and favorable safety profile. PEG-IFNα has several adverse effects as listed below and is contraindicated in patients with decompensated cirrhosis or immune-mediated extrahepatic manifestations of HBV. Overall, due to their convenience and oral route of administration and lower side effect profile, NA therapy is generally preferred (Table 6.5).

PEG-IFNα has a finite treatment course of 48 weeks duration with response evaluated during and following completion of therapy. NA therapy can be stopped after 12 months of therapy in select patient who are non-cirrhotic, are able to achieve stable HBeAg seroconversion, and have undetectable HBV DNA or confirmed loss of HBsAg. Indefinite therapy with NA is recommended

Table 6.5 Approved antiviral therapies for CHB

Drug	Adult dose	Adverse effects	Monitoring/considerations
High barrier against HBV resistance			
Peg-IFNα	180 ug weekly subQ	Flu-like symptoms, fatigue, mood disturbances, cytopenias, autoimmune disorders	CBC (every 1–3 months), TSH every 3 months Contraindicated in decompensated cirrhosis
Entecavir	0.5 or 1 mg daily oral	Lactic acidosis	
Tenofovir disoproxil fumarate (TDF)	300 mg daily oral	Nephropathy, Fanconi syndrome, osteomalacia, lactic acidosis	Creatinine clearance (CrCl) and phosphate at baseline and annually, bone density at baseline
Tenofovir alafenamide (TAF)	25 mg daily oral	Lactic acidosis, less renal and bone disease than TDF	
Low barrier against HBV resistance (therefore not preferred)			
Lamivudine	100 mg daily oral	Pancreatitis, lactic acidosis	
Telbivudine	600 mg daily oral	Elevated creatinine kinase and myopathy, peripheral neuropathy, lactic acidosis	
Adefovir	10 mg daily oral	Acute renal failure, Fanconi syndrome, nephrogenic diabetes insipidus, lactic acidosis	CrCl and phosphate at baseline and annually, consider bone density testing

in adults with HBeAg-negative immune active CHB and those with cirrhosis. Current studies have demonstrated a 61–91% rate of HBV DNA suppression after 2–3 years of continuous therapy with entecavir or tenofovir with normalization of ALT in 66–88% of patients. As stated previously HBsAg loss is rare, occurring in up to about 10% of patients treated with entecavir or tenofovir.

Question 4. What is the recommended follow-up for patients with CHB? Should CHB patients be screened for HCC?

HBV immunologic status changes over time and continued monitoring is required regardless of treatment regimen. Patients who are not candidates for treatment should have periodic assessment of ALT and HBV DNA at 3–6 month intervals. To monitor response to therapy, HBV DNA and ALT are measured every 3 months until undetectable at which time monitoring can be decreased to every 6 months. HBeAg and anti-HBe should be monitored every 6 months in patients who are HBeAg positive. HBsAg should be tested annually.

HCC surveillance is important when caring for patients with CHB. Almost 50% of the mortality in this population is related to HCC and complications related to HCC. Although treatment with antivirals likely lowers the risk of developing HCC, it does not eliminate the risk. Surveillance with AFP and liver ultrasound for HCC should be considered every 6 months for all patients who are HBsAg positive. The AASLD guidelines suggest surveillance is especially important in the following CHB groups:

- Asian men over the age of 40 years old
- Asian women over the age of 50 years

- Patients with cirrhosis
- Africans and African Americans
- Patients with a family history of HCC

Patient Treatment Course

Our patient is a candidate for treatment according to both the ASSLD and EASL criteria outlined above. Treatment with tenofovir alafenamide (TAF) 25 mg orally daily was initiated and well tolerated by the patient. After 6 months of antiviral therapy, HBV DNA viral load was no longer detectable, and AST and ALT had normalized to 16 U/L and 18 U/L, respectively. Renal function remained normal throughout therapy. TAF was continued with plans for repeat HBV serologic testing and renal function annually.

Conclusions

CHB is a complex disease process with global consequences. With screening and early diagnosis, eligible patients may be treated. Current treatments reduce the risk of liver disease progression to cirrhosis and decompensated liver disease. Oral nucleoside/nucleotide analogues tenofovir and entecavir are preferred treatment. Close monitoring and follow-up are important in the care of patients with CHB. The AASLD and EASL guidelines for the treatment of CHB serve as important resource to providers treating patients with CHB.

Further Reading

1. Abara WE, Qaseem A, Schillie S, et al. Hepatitis B vaccination, screening, and linkage to care: best practice advice from the American College of Physicians and the Centers for Disease Control and Prevention. Ann Intern Med. 2017;167:794.
2. Dienstag JL, Hepatitis B. Virus infection. N Engl J Med. 2008;359:1486–500. https://doi.org/10.1056/NEJMra0801644.
3. European Association for the Study of Liver Disease (EASL) 2017 clinical practice guidelines on the management of hepatitis B virus infection. J Hepatol. 2017;67:370–98.
4. Sundaram V, Kowdley K. Management of chronic hepatitis B infection. BMJ. 2015;351:h4263.
5. Terrault, et al. American Association for the Study of Liver Disease (AASLD) guidelines for treatment of chronic hepatitis B. Hepatology. 2016;63:261–83.

Chapter 7
Chronic Hepatitis C

Stanley Martin Cohen

Introduction

Hepatitis C (HCV) is a common viral infection of the liver. It affects approximately 1.6% of the US population. Screening in the appropriate populations is essential as signs and symptoms of the disease are generally absent. In addition, there are multiple new treatments for HCV which are extremely effective and very well tolerated. In this chapter, we describe a case of HCV in an asymptomatic patient. We discuss screening strategies, evaluation of the infection, and treatment options and outcomes.

S. M. Cohen (✉)
Hepatology, Digestive Health Institute, University Hospitals Cleveland Medical Center, Cleveland, OH, USA

Division of Gastroenterology and Liver Disease, Case Western Reserve University School of Medicine, Cleveland, OH, USA
e-mail: stanley.cohen@uhhospitals.org

© Springer Nature Switzerland AG 2019
S. M. Cohen, P. Davitkov (eds.), *Liver Disease*,
https://doi.org/10.1007/978-3-319-98506-0_7

Clinical Case Scenario

A 60-year-old male presents to his primary care provider for a routine physical examination. He has a history of hypertension and borderline diabetes. He denied any past history of surgery. His only medication is an antihypertensive agent. He takes no herbal products or over-the-counter medications. Family history reveals no known history of liver disease. He denied tobacco use. He has never had blood transfusions. He denied tattoos. He has an occasional alcoholic beverage. He denied IV drug use but was somewhat hesitant in answering this question. He is married. They have two adult children. His physical examination is unrevealing except for mild central obesity. Routine labs revealed glucose of 123 mg/dL and an ALT of 45 U/L (with an upper limit of normal of 53 U/L in the lab). His other lab tests including the remainder of the liver panel, CBC, and kidney function were within normal limits. A screening HCV antibody was performed and was positive and he is referred to hepatology clinic. On presentation, the history is essentially unchanged. Physical examination revealed no stigmata of chronic liver disease.

Questions

1. Should this patient have been screened for hepatitis C? What are the current screening guidelines for hepatitis C?
2. With regard to the risk of transmission, what advice should be given to this patient?
3. What additional information should the specialist obtain at this time?
4. What are the treatment options for this patient's hepatitis C and what are the expected cure rates?

Discussion

Question 1. Should this patient have been screened for hepatitis C? What are the current screening guidelines for hepatitis C?

This patient presents with asymptomatic HCV. In fact, this is the most common presentation for this disease. In the absence of symptoms, the clinician is forced to rely on the history for the various risk factors for HCV. These are outlined in Table 7.1 from the American Association for the Study of Liver Diseases-Infectious Disease Society of America (AASLD-IDSA) HCV guidance paper. However, as noted from this table, some of these risk factors include the use of illicit IV drugs and other sensitive information that patients may not want to share with care providers. In addition, care providers may be hesitant to ask such questions. For this

Table 7.1 Recommendations for screening for hepatitis C

Birth cohort born between 1945 and 1965
Injection drug use
Intranasal illicit drug use
Persons on hemodialysis
Persons with percutaneous/parenteral exposures
Healthcare workers with needlestick injuries or mucosal exposures to HCV-infected blood
Children born to HCV-infected mothers
Recipients of blood product transfusions before 1992
Recipients of clotting factors before 1987
Recipients of organ transplants before 1992
Persons who have been incarcerated
Persons with elevated liver function tests
Persons with evidence of liver disease

reason, the CDC put in place the recommendation for a one-time screening of all persons born between 1945 and 1965 (the baby boomers). This birth-cohort screening was felt to be appropriate to identify about 70–80% of all individuals with HCV. In addition, especially with the current opioid epidemic and dramatic increase in tattoos and other parenteral risk factors in the younger population, the older AASLD guidelines can still be quite useful for patients outside of the birth cohort.

It should be noted that there has been debate about the definition of a "normal" ALT level. Many clinicians use their reference normal lab range. However, the AASLD has suggested that normal ALT should be ≤19 U/L in a healthy woman and ≤ 30 U/L in a healthy man. In our patient, he had a "normal" ALT according to the local lab's reference range. However, he would have an elevated ALT according to the AASLD guidelines. This could have been another clue to underlying HCV infection.

Thus, the patient in the case presentation was appropriately screened based on his birth cohort (born between 1945 and 1965). Current screening guidelines use a combination of birth-cohort testing and risk-based testing (especially for those patients born outside of the 1945–1965 time period).

Question 2. With regard to the risk of transmission, what advice should be given to this patient?

The exact duration of this patient's HCV infection is not clear in the absence of a well-defined risk factor. Transmission is uncommon (<5%) to a sexual partner, but it is recommended that sexual partners be tested. Nonsexual household spread is also felt to be uncommon (<5%) through mechanisms such as sharing razorblades and toothbrushes and exposure to blood. Mother-to-child spread is also uncommon (<5%), but the AASLD-IDSA guidelines do recommend screening children of infected mothers. Whether children of infected fathers (with uninfected mothers) need to be tested is much less clear. Casual, nonsexual, spread of HCV is extremely uncommon. There is no evidence to suggest risk of spread through kissing, sharing cups or silverware, or the use of common toilet facilities.

The patient in this case should be told to talk to his wife about getting tested for HCV. He should be told not to share razor blades or toothbrushes with anyone. If he has a blood spill from trauma or an accident, the blood should be viewed as infectious and cleaned up appropriately. He should also consider speaking with his children about getting tested for HCV.

Question 3. What additional information should the specialist obtain at this time?

Upon presentation to the HCV specialist, there are many issues and questions that must be addressed. These include whether the patient has active HCV, what genotype of HCV, how much damage has been done to the liver, is the patient a good HCV treatment candidate, are they at risk for other types of hepatitis, etc.

In this case, the patient was reported to have "normal" LFTs. While most patients with HCV have elevated LFTs, a significant percentage of patients can have active HCV despite normal LFTs. The level of LFTs doesn't actually impact clinical decisions in the diagnosis and treatment of HCV.

When evaluating a patient with a positive HCV antibody test, the next step will be to determine if the infection is active. It must be kept in mind that 15–30% of patients with HCV will clear the infection on their own. In these cases, the initial screening HCV antibody is positive, but the HCV-RNA is negative. For the majority of patients (70–85%) who progress to active chronic HCV, they will have a positive HCV-RNA level. A quantitative assay should be used for this test, because the exact level of HCV-RNA has some therapeutic implications. Certain HCV treatment medications are used for different durations depending on the level of HCV-RNA (see 8- versus 12-week discussion below).

Once the patient is documented to have a positive HCV-RNA, an HCV genotype should be obtained. Depending on the lab used, this may be a separate order or could be a reflex test with the initial HCV-RNA determination. While there have been 11 HCV genotypes described, there are 6 major genotypes. In the USA, genotype 1 accounts for the majority of cases (about 75%), while genotypes 2 and 3 each account for approximately 10% of cases, respectively. Determining the specific genotype in a patient is important as this will potentially alter the treatment regimen. Some genotypes such as genotype 3 are more difficult to treat.

Patients with HCV should be evaluated for other types of liver disease, especially hepatitis and other diseases that could share similar transmission risk factors. Patients should be tested for hepatitis A immunity with hepatitis A total antibody (to decide if vaccines will be warranted). They should also be tested for hepatitis B infection with hepatitis B surface antigen and hepatitis B total core antibody. They should be tested for hepatitis B immunity with hepatitis B surface antibody (to decide if vaccines will be warranted). They should also be tested for HIV. In addition, the initial evaluation by the specialist is a good time to address other potential risk factors for liver disease such as alcohol use and fatty liver disease risk factors.

Determining the stage (amount of scarring) of his liver disease is important for the treatment of his HCV and his general liver care. Using a Metavir score, there are five stages of liver disease. Stage 0 is no fibrosis, stage 1 is mild portal fibrosis without septae, stage 2 is moderate portal fibrosis with septae, stage 3 is bridging fibrosis, and stage 4 is cirrhosis. Determining the stage of fibrosis has implications about the treatment options, as cirrhosis may be treated differently depending on which HCV medication is used. In addition, due to the high cost of the HCV medications, insurance companies often prioritize patients for HCV therapy based on the degree of fibrosis (more fibrosis gets higher priority). Finally, the presence of cirrhosis brings up the possibility of portal hypertension and other complications of liver disease. These patients would need upper endoscopy to be screened for esophageal varices, in addition to appropriate imaging and alpha-fetoprotein (AFP) testing for hepatocellular carcinoma screening.

There are many ways to stage liver disease. The classic test is liver biopsy which is still considered the gold standard. However, there are issues including procedural risk, cost, and even sampling error. For this reason, many investigators have looked at serologic tests of staging as well as radiologic tests of staging. While beyond the scope of this chapter, there are numerous commercially available serologic assays on the market to determine the stage of liver disease (such as FibroSure® and FibroTest®). In general, the accuracy is in the 80% range. While serologic tests alone are the least expensive and easiest way to stage the HCV, many insurance companies do not recognize these alone when considering prioritization for therapy. The most commonly utilized radiologic test uses ultrasound elastography to calculate the stage (such as FibroScan®). The accuracy of these tests is in the 80–90% range. Many practitioners reserve liver biopsy for patients where serologic tests or radiologic tests can't give an accurate answer or when there is significant discrepancy between various tests. For example, in my practice, I use a serologic test as well as an ultrasound elastography. If the results are in agreement, I submit their pre-treatment paperwork using that stage. If there is a significant discrepancy, then I consider a liver biopsy.

Another part of the specialist's role in this case is to determine if the patient is a good HCV treatment candidate. The patient should be assessed for compliance. It should also be determined if they are actively using substances such as alcohol or illicit drugs. Most, but not all, HCV providers require some period of abstinence before embarking on HCV therapy. In addition, some insurance companies mandate a required period of drug and alcohol abstinence (with drug screens) before treatment can be considered.

The patient in this case should be tested for HCV-RNA and genotype. He should have testing for hepatitis A total antibody, hepatitis B surface antigen, hepatitis B total core antibody, hepatitis B surface antibody, and HIV. He should also undergo some type of staging procedure using a noninvasive test(s).

Additional Clinical Information and Test Results and Interpretation

The patient underwent evaluation by the liver specialist and had the following results:
- HCV-RNA: 8,342,278 IU/ml
- HCV genotype: 1b
- Hepatitis A total antibody: Negative
- Hepatitis B surface antigen: Negative
- Hepatitis B core total antibody: Negative
- Hepatitis B surface antibody: Positive
- HIV: Negative
- FibroSure®: Consistent with stage 2, grade 1 disease
- Ultrasound elastography (FibroScan®): Median liver stiffness 8.2 kPa with an IQR of 12%

From this data, the patient has genotype 1b disease with a high viral load. He is not immune to hepatitis A and should be offered vaccinations. He is immune to hepatitis B from prior vaccination. He has stage 2 disease (not cirrhosis) based on both a serologic test and a radiologic test. There is no need to consider a liver biopsy as the staging results are in agreement. He can now be considered for HCV treatment options.

Question 4. What are the treatment options for this patient's hepatitis C, and what are the expected cure rates?

Now that we have all of the baseline information and data on this patient, we can discuss treatment options. This is a rapidly changing field and the treating practitioner must keep up with the various treatment regimens. The best source for up-to-date information on HCV therapy is the AASLD-IDSA HCV guidance paper available at hcvguidelines.org. This is an online document that is constantly updated. It provides guidance on the treatment of all different types of HCV patients.

It should be noted that the insurance company may dictate which therapy the patient receives. Other factors such as drug-drug interaction between the HCV treatments and the patient's medications may influence treatment decisions. Even though the different HCV therapies can vary in terms of number of pills, length of therapy, and sometimes the use of ribavirin, the expected sustained virologic response rates (SVR) or cure rates are all very similar.

The HCV treatment options contain combinations of various direct-acting antiviral agents (DAAs). These include protease inhibitors, NS5A inhibitors, NS5B inhibitors, and occasionally ribavirin. While beyond the scope of this chapter to completely discuss, there can be drug-drug interaction with these various DAAs, and this must be factored into the decision of treatment options.

In my practice, we use a specialty pharmacist to help with HCV therapy. We find them invaluable in these cases. They help determine which therapy is covered by the various insurance companies. They also help with the paperwork such as prior authorization forms. In addition, they help with assessing for drug-drug interactions which might influence therapy decisions. They may also help follow the patients while on therapy.

Based on the patient's clinical information, he is HCV, genotype 1b, treatment-naïve, HCV-RNA > 6,000,000 IU/ml, without cirrhosis. Based on the AASLD-IDSA document, there are many recommended as well as alternative treatment options for this patient. Table 7.2 outlines a representative choice of the recommended options for this particular patient based on the AASLD-IDSA guidance document.

The best choice of HCV therapy in this patient may depend on many factors including cure rates, length of therapy, number of pills daily, potential drug-drug interactions, cost, and insurance preference. In our patient's case, there will be no significant drug-drug interactions to consider in making our decision.

As seen in Table 7.2, there are two recommended treatment options that are 8 weeks in length. However, because our patient has an HCV-RNA > 6,000,000 IU/ml, he is actually not a candidate for 8 weeks of ledipasvir/sofosbuvir. His only 8-week option would be glecaprevir/pibrentasvir.

All of the recommended regimens in Table 7.2 are one pill daily, except for glecaprevir/pibrentasvir which requires three pills daily.

Table 7.2 AASLD-IDSA recommended regimens for HCV treatment in a treatment-naïve, non-cirrhotic patient with HCV genotype 1b infection

Recommended regimen	Duration
Daily fixed-dose combination of glecaprevir (300 mg)/pibrentasvir (120 mg)	8 weeks
Daily fixed-dose combination of ledipasvir (90 mg)/sofosbuvir (400 mg)	12 weeks
Daily fixed-dose combination of ledipasvir (90 mg)/sofosbuvir (400 mg) for patients who are non-black and HIV-uninfected and whose HCV-RNA level is <6 million IU/mL	8 weeks
Daily fixed-dose combination of sofosbuvir (400 mg)/velpatasvir (100 mg)	12 weeks
Daily fixed-dose combination of elbasvir (50 mg)/grazoprevir (100 mg)	12 weeks

Table 7.3 SVR rates for different HCV treatment regimens (and their supporting registration study names)

Elbasvir + graz-eprevir (C-EDGE)	Sofosbuvir + ledi-pasvir (ION1/3) (12 or 8 weeks, if eligible for 8 week course)	Glecaprevir + pibren-tasvir (ENDURANCE-1)	Sofosbuvir + vel-patasvir (Astral-1)
95%	97%	99%	98%

The sustained virologic response rate (SVR) is defined as an undetectable HCV-RNA 12 weeks (SVR12) and/or 24 weeks (SVR24) after the completion of the therapy. This is considered a cure of the infection. While the FDA now recognizes SVR12 as a cure, many clinicians still follow for SVR12 and SVR24. As shown in Table 7.3, the SVR rates are very high (95–99%) for our patient regardless of which recommended regimen is used.

Patient Treatment Course

Because there was no particularly pressing reason to choose one regimen over another, I had the specialty pharmacist submit his insurance paperwork. The insurance's preferred option was 12 weeks of ledipasvir/sofosbuvir. The patient was counseled on the importance of medication compliance. He was told of the potential adverse effects (generally limited to mild headache and fatigue).

He took the regimen for the 12 week period without difficulty. His labs were stable on treatment. His HCV-RNA was already undetectable within 4 weeks of starting the treatment. His end-of-treatment, 1-month post-treatment, 3-months post-treatment, and 6-months post-treatment liver function tests were normal, and his HCV-RNA was undetectable at each of those same timepoints. He thus obtained an SVR and was cured of his HCV infection.

Given the fact that he had mild fibrosis (stage 2), he was discharged from the liver clinic and sent back to his primary provider. There are no recommendations for follow-up HCV-RNA testing, unless he were to encounter new risk factors and/or new exposures.

If he had had cirrhosis (stage 4), it must be noted that he would be cured of his HCV infection but not his cirrhosis. Generally, we continue to follow those patients in our liver clinic as they could still be at risk for complications of cirrhosis such as decompensation, liver cancer development, or the formation of esophageal varices.

Conclusions

Hepatitis C is a common disease and very specific screening recommendations exist. The most important is one-time screening for those born between 1945 and 1965. While sexual and household transmission is uncommon, patients and their contacts should be cautioned about the risk factors. HCV treaters should see the patient and complete the full pre-treatment evaluation. Specialty pharmacists can be very helpful in the process of pre-treatment evaluation and helping to obtain therapy. There are many, very effective treatment options for HCV with cure rates in the 95–99% range. The best guidance document is the online AASLD-IDSA recommendations available at hcvguidelines.org.

Further Reading

1. Afdhal N, et al. Ledipasvir and sofosbuvir for untreated HCV genotype 1 infection (ION-1 study). N Engl J Med. 2014;370:1889–98.
2. American Association for the Study of Liver Disease/Infectious Disease Society of America (AASLD-IDSA). HCV guidance: recommendations

for testing, managing, and treating hepatitis C. http://hcvguidelines.org. Accessed 9 Nov 2017.

3. CDC guidelines on HCV screening. http://www.cdc.gov/nchhstp/news-room/HepTestingRecsPressRelease2012.html. Accessed 23 May 2012.

4. Feld JJ, et al. Sofosbuvir and velpatasvir for HCV genotype 1,2,4,5, and 6 infection. N Engl J Med. 2015;373:2599–607.

5. Kowdley KV, et al. Ledipasvir and sofosbuvir for 8 or 12 weeks for chronic HCV without cirrhosis (ION-3 study). N Engl J Med. 2014;370:1879–88.

6. Rockstroh JK, et al. Efficacy and safety of grazoprevir and elbasvir in patients with hepatitis C virus and HIV co-infection (C-EDGE Co-Infection): a non-randomised, open label trial. The Lancet HIV. 2015;2:e319–27.

7. Zeuzem S, et al. ENDURANCE-1: A phase 3 evaluation of the efficacy and safety of 8- versus 12-week treatment with glecaprevir/Pibrentasvir in HCV genotype 1 infected patients with or without HIV-1 co-infection and without cirrhosis. Presented as a poster at AASLD 2016, Boston MA.

Chapter 8
Nonalcoholic Fatty Liver Disease

Nael N. Haddad, Amandeep Singh, Mazyar Malakouti, and Naim Alkhouri

Introduction

Nonalcoholic fatty liver disease (NAFLD) is defined as the presence of excessive fat accumulation in the liver in individuals without significant alcohol consumption or other etiologies of chronic liver disease. It is the most common cause of chronic liver disease in the United States and is rapidly becoming the most common indication for liver transplantation. NAFLD encompasses a broad spectrum of diseases, ranging from simple

N. N. Haddad
University of Texas Health San Antonio, Department of Internal
Medicine, San Antonio, TX, USA

A. Singh
Cleveland Clinic, Department of Gastroenterology and Hepatology,
Cleveland, OH, USA

M. Malakouti
University of Texas Health San Antonio, Department
of Gastroenterology, San Antonio, TX, USA

N. Alkhouri (✉)
University of Texas Health San Antonio, Department
of Gastroenterology, San Antonio, TX, USA

Texas Liver Institute, San Antonio, TX, USA
e-mail: alkhouri@txliver.com

© Springer Nature Switzerland AG 2019
S. M. Cohen, P. Davitkov (eds.), *Liver Disease*,
https://doi.org/10.1007/978-3-319-98506-0_8

steatosis or nonalcoholic fatty liver (NAFL), progressing through nonalcoholic steatohepatitis (NASH) and advanced fibrosis, to cirrhosis and end-stage liver disease. Most patients with NAFLD are asymptomatic and are often diagnosed incidentally. They often present with elevated liver enzymes on routine blood work or with incidental findings of hepatic steatosis (HS) on imaging studies performed for other reasons. In this chapter we will discuss the epidemiology, natural history, diagnosis modalities, assessment of disease severity, and the available treatment options for NAFLD.

Clinical Scenario

A 50-year-old male presents to his primary care physician for a regular follow-up visit. The patient has a past medical history of type 2 diabetes mellitus (T2DM), dyslipidemia, and essential hypertension (HTN) but denies any significant past surgical history. He has been on the same medications for the past 2 years without any change, including lisinopril, simvastatin, and metformin. He denies the use of any over-the-counter medications or herbal products. He drinks 3–4 cans of beer per week but denies smoking cigarettes or use of illicit drugs. His physical exam is notable for central obesity with a body mass index (BMI) of 33 kg/m^2. During his last visit, routine laboratory tests were ordered, along with abdominal ultrasound (US) due to the suspicion of a kidney stone. His laboratory tests were normal except for a mild elevation of aspartate aminotransferase (AST) and alanine aminotransferase (ALT) (86 U/L and 70 U/L, respectively). Abdominal US revealed a small 4 mm stone in the right kidney. Incidental finding of hyperechoic texture of the liver consistent with steatosis was also noted. The patient was scheduled for a follow-up visit and a viral hepatitis panel along with repeat liver enzymes was ordered. On the next visit, the patient's hepatitis panel was negative, and his liver enzymes were essentially unchanged from the prior visit. Due to the presence of abnormal liver enzymes and steatosis seen on ultrasound, a diagnosis of NAFLD was considered.

Questions

1. Is NAFLD common and why do we need to diagnose it?
2. What are the risk factors associated with NAFLD?
3. How do we diagnose a patient with suspected NAFLD?
4. How can we assess the severity of the disease?
5. What are the available treatment options for NAFLD?

Discussion

Question 1. Is NAFLD common and why do we need to diagnose it?

NAFLD is considered the hepatic manifestation of the metabolic syndrome (MetS). Due to the worldwide rise in the incidence of diabetes and obesity, the prevalence of NAFLD has increased significantly. NAFLD has become the most common chronic liver disorder in Western industrialized countries. The global prevalence of NAFLD was found to be around 25%, with the highest prevalence rates in the Middle East (32%) and lowest in Africa (14%).

Patients with NAFLD can be broadly classified into two major subtypes: the relatively benign nonalcoholic fatty liver (NAFL) or simple steatosis and the aggressive nonalcoholic steatohepatitis (NASH) which includes the presence of steatosis and necro-inflammation with or without fibrosis. The majority of NAFLD patients have a benign disease course and are classified as having NAFL. A subset of individuals develops NASH and can progress to develop advanced fibrosis, cirrhosis, hepatocellular carcinoma (HCC), and end-stage liver disease requiring liver transplantation. Currently NASH is the second most common cause of liver transplantation after hepatitis C and is predicted to be the number one indication in the near future as more hepatitis C patients are getting treated with highly effective antiviral medications. Furthermore, it is important to point out that many patients with cryptogenic cirrhosis could have what is considered to be "burned-out" NASH as these patients seem to have a high prevalence of the same metabolic risk factors including T2DM, obesity, and MetS.

Patients with NAFLD and NASH in particular have increased risk of overall mortality when compared to control population without NAFLD, as well as liver-, cardiovascular-, and malignancy-related deaths. The most common cause of death in NAFLD patients seems to be cardiovascular disease (CVD), independent of other metabolic comorbidities, followed by cancer and liver-related mortality. HCC is the most common form of liver cancer and is the third leading cause of cancer-related death in the world. Currently, NAFLD is considered to be the third most common cause of HCC in United States, likely due to the large number of patients diagnosed with this condition. The incidence of NAFLD-related HCC is increasing given the growing epidemic of obesity. Some studies have also demonstrated that HCC can potentially develop in NAFLD patients even in the absence of cirrhosis.

Question 2. What are the risk factors associated with NAFLD?

The association between MetS and NAFLD has been strongly established. Obesity, T2DM, and dyslipidemia are the most recognized metabolic risk factors for developing NAFLD. Of all the individual components of MetS, obesity has the strongest association with NAFLD. Studies have shown a prevalence of NAFLD in up to 70% of obese patients and up to 90% in patients with severe obesity undergoing bariatric surgery.

Hyperglycemia and insulin resistance (IR) characterize T2DM. Insulin resistance plays an important role in the pathogenesis of NAFLD, which explains the strong connection between these two disorders. Defective insulin signaling leads to inefficient suppression of gluconeogenesis in the liver and the impairment of glucose uptake in muscle cells and adipose tissues. In adipose tissues, impaired insulin signaling promotes lipolysis resulting in an elevation of levels of circulating fatty acids and increased uptake by liver. This, along with an increase in de novo liver lipogenesis caused by insulin resistance, contributes to the development of NAFLD in approximately 75% of patients with T2DM.

Dyslipidemia, especially high serum triglyceride levels and low serum high-density lipoprotein levels, is commonly seen in NAFLD patients with an estimated prevalence of 50%. Other conditions including polycystic ovarian syndrome (PCOS), hypothyroidism, obstructive sleep apnea (OSA), hypopituitarism, hypogonadism, and psoriasis have also been associated with NAFLD.

Because of the strong relationship between NAFLD and MetS, it is recommended that patients with incidental hepatic steatosis detected on imaging should be assessed for metabolic risk factors such as T2DM and dyslipidemia, even without any signs or symptoms of liver disease.

On the other hand, the American Association for the Study of Liver Diseases (AASLD) does not advise at this time to routinely screen for NAFLD in high-risk groups because of the lack of sufficient evidence related to diagnostic modalities, treatment options, long-term benefits, and effectiveness of screening. This is in contrast to recommendations by the European Association for the Study of the Liver (EASL) that recommends screening for NAFLD by liver enzymes and/or ultrasound in subjects with obesity or MetS. It is our opinion that screening will be adopted by practice guidelines once new effective treatments for advanced NAFLD outside of lifestyle modifications are approved.

Question 3. How do we diagnose a patient with suspected NAFLD?

Most patients with NAFLD are asymptomatic and are often diagnosed incidentally when liver enzymes are noted to be abnormal or evidence of HS is seen on imaging performed for other reasons.

The diagnosis of NAFLD requires the following:

1. Evidence of HS by imaging or histology
2. No significant alcohol consumption
3. No evidence of other chronic liver diseases or conditions that can cause HS

There are many diseases that are associated with secondary HS, and it is important to rule out the different causes of steatosis before narrowing down the diagnosis to NAFLD. Chronic liver diseases such as Wilson disease; chronic hepatitis C genotype 3 infection; certain inborn errors of metabolism, like abetalipoproteinemia; and conditions such as starvation and parenteral nutrition are associated with varying degrees of HS. Alcoholic liver disease is a very common and important cause of secondary HS and can be indistinguishable from NAFLD on liver biopsy. This is why it is crucial to rule out excess alcohol intake before making a diagnosis of NAFLD. Significant alcohol consumption is defined as >21 drinks per week (3 drinks per day) in men and > 14 drinks per week (2 drinks per day) in women.

When evaluating a patient with suspected NAFLD, it is also important to focus on medication history, as there are several drugs associated with secondary HS including corticosteroids, amiodarone, methotrexate, valproate, and antiretroviral agents for HIV.

Serum aminotransferases are usually abnormal in patients with suspected NAFLD. The increase is usually moderate, 1–4 times the upper limit of normal. Aminotransferase levels do not reflect the extent of the disease, and a low to normal ALT level does not guarantee the absence of underlying HS. Serological evaluation in patients with suspected NAFLD can sometimes uncover laboratory abnormalities commonly associated with other liver disorders. For example, mild elevation in serum ferritin is common in NALFD and does not necessarily indicate hepatic iron overload; it might, however, impact disease prognosis. It is important to mention that when elevated serum ferritin and transferrin saturation are present in patients with suspected NAFLD, hereditary hemochromatosis should be excluded.

The presence of low titers of autoantibodies, such as anti-smooth muscle and antinuclear antibodies, is also common in NAFLD patients but not considered to have any clinical consequence. However, the presence of such antibodies in high titers, especially in conjunction with an increase in immunoglobulins, requires a liver biopsy in order to exclude autoimmune hepatitis. Table 8.1 provides a list of laboratory tests that we commonly obtain in our patients with suspected NAFLD to rule out other etiologies for elevation in liver enzymes/HS and to assess for comorbidities.

Only histological examination of the liver can confirm the diagnosis of NAFLD, which is why liver biopsy is considered the "gold standard." However, expense, possible complications associated with the procedure, and the need of expertise for interpretation limit its use on a large scale. Biopsy is performed only in selected patients, those who are at high risk of having steatohepatitis or advanced fibrosis, and when the etiology of HS/elevated liver enzymes or the presence of other chronic liver diseases cannot be excluded.

Table 8.1 Commonly used laboratory tests in patients with NAFLD

Laboratory test	Other etiologies/comorbidities
Chronic viral hepatitis panel	Hepatitis C and B
Smooth muscle antibody (SMA), antinuclear antibody (ANA), anti-mitochondrial antibody (AMA)	Autoimmune liver disease (autoimmune hepatitis and primary biliary cholangitis)
Alpha-1 antitrypsin level/phenotype	Alpha-1 antitrypsin deficiency
Iron, TIBC, ferritin	Hereditary hemochromatosis
Ceruloplasmin	Wilson disease
Thyroid-stimulating hormone (TSH)	Hypothyroidism
Lipid panel	Dyslipidemia
HbA1C	Pre-diabetes, T2DM

Question 4. How can we assess the severity of NAFLD?

Based on histological features, NAFLD can be divided into three major categories:

1. NAFL (nonalcoholic fatty liver): Presence of >5% of HS without significant necro-inflammation or fibrosis
2. NASH: (nonalcoholic steatohepatitis): Presence of >5% of HS with inflammation and hepatocyte injury in the form of ballooning with or without fibrosis
3. NASH cirrhosis: Presence of cirrhosis with current or previous evidence of steatosis

The majority of NAFLD patients do not progress to cirrhosis and are broadly classified as having NAFL; however, the remaining patients with NAFLD will have NASH that can potentially lead to advanced fibrosis, cirrhosis, HCC, and end-stage liver disease necessitating a liver transplantation.

NASH is considered as a histological entity, and liver biopsy is required for its diagnosis. However, recent data have demonstrated clearly that liver fibrosis is the most important prognostic factor in predicting liver-related outcomes in patients with NAFLD. Therefore, the identification of those patients with advanced fibrosis related to NAFLD is a high priority. Luckily, there are several noninvasive tools for assessment of advanced fibrosis in NAFLD that have been validated in different populations including serum biomarkers/clinical variables put together in formulas to provide fibrosis scores and imaging modalities.

NAFLD fibrosis score (NFS) is a tool commonly used for assessing advanced fibrosis. It is calculated using six routinely measured variables including age, BMI, blood glucose levels, platelet count, albumin, and AST/ALT ratio. By setting a low cutoff (<-1.455), advanced fibrosis can be excluded with high accuracy (negative predictive value of 93%), while a high cutoff threshold (>0.676) provides accurate detection of advanced fibrosis (positive predictive value of 90%). Fibrosis-4 (FIB-4) index is another algorithm for detecting advanced fibrosis, and it is based on platelet count, age, AST, and ALT. Other indices including AST to platelet ratio index (APRI) and AST/ALT ratio are inferior for predicting advanced fibrosis when compared to NFS and the FIB-4 index.

Elastography imaging modalities-* are used to measure the stiffness of the liver as a noninvasive method to estimate liver fibrosis. Studies have shown strong correlation between liver stiffness measurement (LSM) and the degree of fibrosis in NAFLD. Both US and MRI-based techniques are available to quantify the degree of stiffness in the liver.

US elastography techniques have demonstrated very promising results for assessing liver fibrosis in NAFLD. Vibration-controlled transient elastography (VCTE) marketed as FibroScan® is FDA-approved. FibroScan® uses a modified ultrasound probe to measure the velocity of a shear wave created by a vibratory source. This velocity is converted mathematically into LSM depicted in kilopascals (kPa). Using the cutoff points of approximately 7–10 kPa has reasonable accuracy for ruling out and ruling in advanced fibrosis, respectively. Unfortunately,

LSM results could be unreliable in severely obese patients with BMI of more than 40 kg/m2. MRI elastography can measure liver stiffness with potentially higher accuracy and the advantage of being able to assess stiffness over the entire liver. However, due to high cost and limited availability, VCTE might be more favorable for routine clinical use. Figure 8.1 provides the

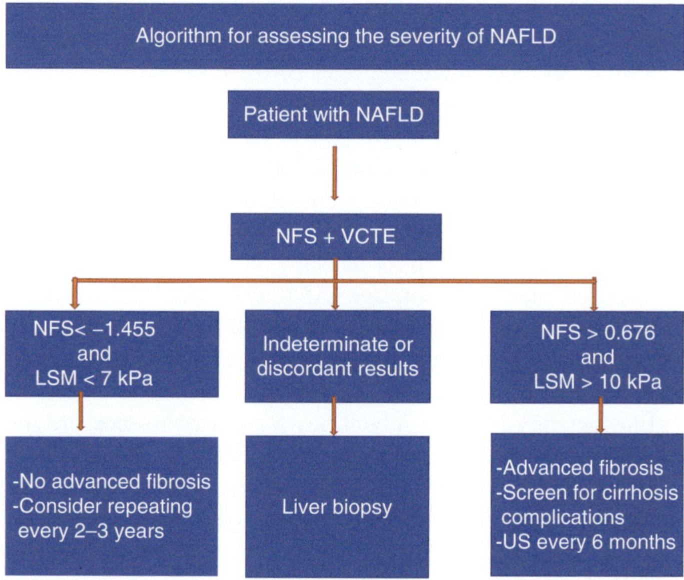

Fig. 8.1 Noninvasive assessment of NAFLD severity through the use of NAFLD fibrosis score (NFS) and FibroScan®-based vibration-controlled transient elastography (VCTE). Scenario 1: NFS score of <1.455 and liver stiffness measurement (LSM) of <7 kPa → low probability of having significant fibrosis, recommend weight loss through lifestyle modifications, and consider repeating the tests every 2–3 years. Scenario 2: Indeterminate results include patients with NFS score between 0.676 and 1.445 or patients with LSM between 7 and 10. Discordant results indicate that NFS and LSM provided contradictory results (e.g., high NFS with low LSM) →. Consider a liver biopsy to determine the presence of NASH and the fibrosis stage. Scenario 3: NFS score of >0.676 and LSM of >10 kPa → likely to have advanced fibrosis, and screening for cirrhosis complications is recommended. Consider referral to clinical trials with anti-fibrotic agents

approach that we utilize in our clinic to noninvasively assess the severity of liver fibrosis in NAFLD patients.

Question 5. What are the available treatment options for NAFLD?

Lifestyle Modifications

Currently there are no approved pharmacological treatments for NAFLD, and lifestyle modifications to induce weight loss through diet and exercise remain the cornerstone of therapy.

Obesity plays an important role in the pathophysiology of NAFLD, which is why weight loss is the first-line therapy. Current evidence suggests that a loss of 3–5% of body weight improves HS; a loss of 5–7% reduces inflammatory activity and other features of NASH, and a loss of $\geq 10\%$ may result in resolution of NASH and regression of fibrosis. Based on these data, we recommend 10% total body weight loss to our patients.

There are not any specific recommendations regarding the type of diet that may improve or halt disease progression in NAFLD; however, data suggest that the Mediterranean diet may have the most benefit for reducing HS and preventing CVD. More recently, several studies have shown beneficial effects of coffee drinking in patients with NAFLD, and, therefore, we recommend two cups of black coffee a day to our patients. When counseling patients about their diet, it is important to address that they should not consume heavy amounts of alcohol.

Exercise alone may prevent or decrease HS. One study showed that patients maintaining more than 150 min/week of physical activity or increasing their activity level by more than 60 min/week had greater reduction in serum aminotransferases, independent of weight loss when compared to individuals who were less active. Unfortunately, the majority of patients with NAFLD are not able to achieve and sustain the recommended weight loss and exercise goals.

Pharmacological Treatment

Several pharmacological agents have been evaluated for treatment of NASH, but still there are no FDA-approved medications. Medications that are used with a goal of improving liver histology/disease are generally reserved for those with biopsy-proven NASH and fibrosis.

Because of the association of IR with NAFLD, insulin sensitizers have been widely studied for NASH. Data regarding metformin have not been consistent. Initially, the use of metformin showed a reduction in IR along with improvement in ALT levels; however, recent meta-analyses have shown no improvement in liver histology. Currently metformin is not recommended as a treatment option for these patients. In a large randomized controlled trial, pioglitazone 30 mg/day improved histological features of NASH such as steatosis, inflammation, hepatocyte ballooning, and resolution of NASH. However, the safety of using pioglitazone remains an issue. Weight gain is the most common side effect with pioglitazone treatment, but other more serious side effects have been reported including osteoporosis and potentially bladder cancer. The AASLD suggests that pioglitazone could be considered for treatment of biopsy-proven NASH (with or without T2DM) after discussing the risks and benefits with each patient and recommended against its use for NAFLD patients without biopsy-proven NASH given the issues surrounding its safety and efficacy. The glucagon-like peptide-1 (GLP-1) agonist, liraglutide, might have beneficial effects in NASH patients, but large studies are needed before we can recommend its use for this indication.

Vitamin E is an antioxidant that has been investigated for the treatment of NASH as oxidative stress plays a major role in hepatocyte injury and disease progression. Vitamin E at a dose of 800 IU/day improved histological features of NASH including steatosis, inflammation, ballooning, and the NAFLD activity score in nondiabetic patients. However, there have been some concerns regarding the long-term use of vitamin E as it was associated with increased all-cause mortality, incidence of hemorrhagic stroke, and risk of prostate cancer in different studies. Vitamin E can be considered as a treatment option in nondiabetic patients with biopsy-proven NASH.

Novel Investigational Drugs

Several agents with novel mechanisms of action are in late-stage development as treatments for NASH and liver fibrosis. These include elafibranor, a dual peroxisome proliferator-activated receptor alpha/delta (PPAR-α/δ) agonist that plays a role in hepatocyte fatty acid metabolism; obeticholic acid, a potent farnesoid X receptor agonist that reduces liver fat and fibrosis; cenicriviroc, an antagonist of C-C chemokine receptor types 2 and 5 (CCR2/CCR5) which mediate interactions driving inflammation and fibrosis; and selonsertib, an inhibitor of apoptosis signal-regulating kinase-1 (ASK-1), which typically promotes hepatic inflammation and fibrosis. We are optimistic that the first FDA-approved drugs for NASH will become available around 2020.

Patient Treatment Course

Our patient underwent further evaluation. His serologies were unrevealing for any other causes of liver disease. He underwent NFS and VCTE testing which revealed low scores consistent with no evidence of advanced fibrosis. He was told to aggressively work on the various lifestyle modifications and risk factors for fatty liver disease. He was told to keep his alcohol intake to a minimum. He was vaccinated against hepatitis A and hepatitis B. He will follow up in the clinic to assess his clinical course and consider repeat staging of his fatty liver disease in 2–3 years.

Conclusion/Summary

NAFLD is the most common cause of chronic liver disease in the United States and represents a worldwide public health burden. Clinicians should have a high index of suspicion to diagnose NAFLD because the disease is clinically silent until late stages. There are no FDA-approved medications for treatment, and lifestyle modifications are still considered to be the only effective option. Unfortunately, the current treatment options have limited efficacy, but the future seems to be bright as new NASH-specific therapies with promising results are being studied.

Further Readings

1. Adams LA, Lymp JF, St Sauver J, et al. The natural history of non-alcoholic fatty liver disease: a population-based cohort study. Gastroenterology. 2005;129:113–21.
2. Angulo P, Kleiner DE, Dam-Larsen S, et al. Liver fibrosis, but no other histologic features, is associated with long-term outcomes of patients with nonalcoholic fatty liver disease. Gastroenterology. 2015;149(2):389–97.
3. Chalasani N, Younossi Z, Lavine JE, et al. The diagnosis and management of nonalcoholic fatty liver disease: practice guidance from the American Association for the Study of Liver Diseases. Hepatology. 2018;67(1):328–57.
4. Cusi K, Orsak B, Bril F, et al. Long-term pioglitazone treatment for patients with nonalcoholic steatohepatitis and prediabetes or type 2 diabetes mellitus: a randomized trial. Ann Intern Med. 2016;165:305–15.
5. EASL-EASD-EASO clinical practice guidelines for the management of non-alcoholic fatty liver disease. J Hepatol. 2016;64(6):1388–402.
6. Mittal S, El-Serag HB, Sada YH, et al. Hepatocellular carcinoma in the absence of cirrhosis in United States veterans is associated with nonalcoholic fatty liver disease. Clin Gastroenterol Hepatol. 2016;14(1):31.e1.

7. Sanyal AJ, Chalasani N, Kowdley KV, et al. Pioglitazone, vitamin E, or placebo for non- alcoholic steatohepatitis. N Engl J Med. 2010;362:1675–85.
8. Tapper EB, Challies T, Nasser I, et al. The performance of vibration controlled transient elastography in a US cohort of patients with nonalcoholic fatty liver disease. Am J Gastroenterol. 2016;111:677–84.
9. Vilar-Gomez E, Martinez-Perez Y, Calzadilla-Bertot L, et al. Weight loss through lifestyle modification significantly reduces features of nonalcoholic steatohepatitis. Gastroenterology. 2015;149:367–78.
10. Younossi ZM, Koenig AB, Abdelatif D, et al. Global epidemiology of nonalcoholic fatty liver disease-meta-analytic assessment of prevalence, incidence, and outcomes. Hepatology. 2016;64(1):73–84.

Chapter 9
Liver Disease and Pregnancy

Lydia Aye and Tram Tran

Introduction

Recognition of normal and abnormal liver tests and physiology in pregnancy is essential. Rarely does a pregnant woman experience severe liver disease during her pregnancy, but it is important to recognize these patients to reduce morbidity and mortality for the mother and infant. We will discuss liver disease in a pregnant patient and liver diseases unique to pregnancy.

Clinical Case Scenario

A 28-year-old Asian woman (G_1P_0) is 20 weeks pregnant and presents to your office for abnormal liver enzymes. She has no other medical problems. She occasionally drank 1–2 glasses of wine but stopped when she found out she was pregnant. She denies smoking tobacco or using illicit drugs. She denies any

L. Aye
Division of Gastroenterology and Hepatology, Loma Linda University, Loma Linda, CA, USA

T. Tran (✉)
South Bay Gastroenterology, Torrance, CA, USA
e-mail: Tram.Tran@cshs.org

© Springer Nature Switzerland AG 2019
S. M. Cohen, P. Davitkov (eds.), *Liver Disease*,
https://doi.org/10.1007/978-3-319-98506-0_9

family history of liver diseases. Her pregnancy has been uneventful, and she had some nausea and vomiting during her first trimester, but that has since improved. Her labs reveal a normal CBC and renal function. Her liver tests are remarkable for AST 100 U/L, ALT 120 U/L, alkaline phosphatase U/L, and total bilirubin 0.5 mg/dL. Right upper quadrant ultrasound revealed a normal liver with no biliary ductal dilatation.

Questions

1. What work-up should a pregnant patient undergo for abnormal liver tests?
2. What tests can a pregnant patient undergo?
3. What work-up should a pregnant patient with suspected acute viral hepatitis undergo?
4. What treatments are available for patients with chronic viral hepatitis? When is it appropriate to treat chronic viral hepatitis in a pregnant patient?
5. What liver diseases are unique to pregnancy? In what trimester do these diseases usually occur?

Discussion

Question 1. What work-up should a pregnant patient undergo for abnormal liver tests?

Abnormal liver tests occur in approximately 3–5% of pregnant women. Physiological changes due to pregnancy can cause changes to liver tests that are in fact physiologically normal. Most of the liver tests remain the same during pregnancy except

Table 9.1 Normal changes in liver lab tests during pregnancy

Test	Change in pregnancy
Hemoglobin	Decrease
AST	No change
Alt	No change
Alkaline phosphatase	Increase
Total bilirubin	No change
Albumin	Decrease

for alkaline phosphatase and albumin (see Table 9.1). Alkaline phosphatase is increased in pregnancy because it is produced by the placenta. Albumin levels appear low due to hemodilution. Other abnormalities, including elevated transaminases and bilirubin, should not be caused by pregnancy and do require further investigation. The initial work-up for a pregnant woman with abnormal liver test should be the same as with any nonpregnant patient. A complete history, physical exam, and serological testing should be based on clinical presentation.

The patient in the case presentation has mildly elevated alkaline phosphatase, which is probably physiologically normal. However, her elevated transaminases are not normal and require further evaluation.

Question 2. What tests can a pregnant patient undergo?

Lab work and serological testing are safe in a pregnant patient. Imaging may be needed in a pregnant patient to evaluate the liver, liver vasculature, or biliary system. The initial imaging test should be an ultrasound with or without Doppler. Ultrasound uses sound waves, not ionizing radiation, and has not been shown to have any adverse fetal effects. If ultrasound is indeterminate, CT or MRI without gadolinium can be considered. Radiation exposure has been associated with fetal growth restriction and microcephaly, but the risk does not appear to be increased if the exposure is ≤5 rad. The greatest risk of radiation is exposure during 8–15 weeks of gestation. An abdominal x-ray has a fetal exposure of approximately 100 mrad. CT scan of the abdomen has a fetal exposure of approximately 3.5 rad. Although intravenous contrast agents have not been shown to be teratogenic in animal studies, there is an association with neonatal hypothyroidism in association with iodinated contrast exposure during pregnancy. MRI with contrast is not recommended because gadolinium crosses the placenta and is excreted by fetal kidneys into the amniotic fluid. The excreted gadolinium can remain in the amniotic fluid for a long period of time which exposes the fetus' pulmonary and gastrointestinal to potential injury.

Question 3. What work-up should a pregnant patient with suspected acute viral hepatitis undergo?

Pregnant patients with suspected acute viral hepatitis should be tested for common causes of acute liver injury. Causes of acute liver injury include hepatitis A (HAV), hepatitis B (HBV), hepatitis C (HCV), hepatitis E (HEV), and herpes simplex virus (HSV).

Acute HAV is the most common cause of acute viral hepatitis. HAV accounts for 20–40% of cases of adult viral hepatitis in the Western world but is infrequently reported in pregnant patients. The serologic test for acute hepatitis A is the HAV IgM antibody. There have been no reported mortalities of mother or baby from acute HAV infection during pregnancy. The Centers for Disease Control and Prevention (CDC) recommends HAV immunoglobulin treatment for the neonate if the maternal HAV infection occurs within 2 weeks of delivery.

Acute HBV can occur during pregnancy but is much more likely to be chronic HBV in a pregnant patient. Acute HBV can be tested for with hepatitis B surface antigen (HBsAg) and hepatitis B core antibody IgM (HBcIgM). Chronic HBV can be tested for with HBsAg and HBc total antibody. Chronic HBV in pregnancy is discussed below.

Acute HCV can also rarely occur during pregnancy but is again much more likely to be a pregnant woman with chronic HCV. Acute and chronic HCV can be tested for with HCV antibody and HCV-RNA. Chronic HCV in pregnancy is discussed below.

Acute HEV in pregnancy can be associated with rapid acute liver failure with median time from presentation to death or transplant or recovery of 5 days. HEV infection is rare in the USA and Europe but is more common in Pakistan, India, and Mexico. Serologies should be completed in a pregnant patient presenting with acute hepatitis, especially one who has traveled recently to endemic countries, to prepare for possible progression to acute liver failure and possible evaluation for liver transplantation. There is no antiviral treatment for acute HEV.

Acute HSV hepatitis is very rare but should be suspected in a patient who presents with fever, upper respiratory infection symptoms, or anicteric, severe hepatitis. Acute HSV hepatitis is most prevalent in immunosuppressed patients or during pregnancy. The diagnosis can be difficult to make, and HSV PCR should be performed when HSV hepatitis is suspected. Treatment is empiric acyclovir if HSV hepatitis is suspected. Early initiation of treatment (even before the diagnosis is made) has better outcomes then delayed treatment of a confirmed infection. Prophylaxis with acyclovir is recommended by the American College of Obstetrics and Gynecology at 36 weeks of pregnancy to prevent HSV recurrence and prevent vertical transmission in women with previous infection.

Question 4. What treatments are available for patients with chronic viral hepatitis? When is it appropriate to treat chronic viral hepatitis in a pregnant patient?

Hepatitis B (HBV) and hepatitis C (HCV) can cause acute and chronic viral hepatitis. There are effective treatments available for chronic HBV and HCV; however, approximately 65–90% of infected people do not know they are infected.

Chronic HBV affects more than 350 million people worldwide. Screening for HBV is universal for pregnant women in the USA. Vertical transmission from mother to child remains an important cause of HBV transmission. The majority of vertical transmission occurs at delivery. The combination of hepatitis B immunoglobulin and vaccination of infant within 12 h of birth has reduced the rate of perinatal transmission from >90% to <10%. Failure of prevention of transmission occurs in approximately 10% of infants with mothers with high viral load >200,000 IU/mL. Current guidelines recommend antiviral therapy in the third trimester for women with an HBV DNA >200,000 IU/mL to prevent perinatal transmission. Telbivudine and tenofovir are rated pregnancy category B and lamivudine is category C by the FDA. Tenofovir has a high resistance barrier with no resistance identified to date after up to 6 years of monotherapy for chronic HBV. Per the AASLD guidelines, tenofovir is the preferred therapy in pregnancy.

The CDC recommends that any woman pregnant with a known or suspected risk factor for chronic HCV should be tested for HCV infection. Current guidelines recommend that women of reproductive age with known chronic HCV be treated with antiviral therapy before considering pregnancy if possible, but treatment during pregnancy is not recommended at this time.

Question 5. What liver diseases are unique to pregnancy? In what trimester do these diseases usually occur?

There are several liver diseases unique to pregnancy (Table 9.2). These diseases usually resolve with delivery. Gestational age of the pregnancy is important in making the diagnosis and can help determine what evaluation the patient will need.

Hyperemesis gravidarum (HG) occurs during the first trimester of the pregnancy and resolves by 12–20 weeks of gestation. HG is persistent vomiting with >5% weight loss of prepregnancy body weight, dehydration, and ketosis. Liver test abnormalities are common in HG. There is usually a mild elevation of liver enzymes, but levels more than 20 times the upper limit of normal are rarely reported. Elevated bilirubin and synthetic dysfunction are uncommon in HG. HG has been associated with small for gestational age babies, low birth weight, preterm birth, and poor 5 min Apgar scores. Treatment is supportive care, and hospitalization is infrequently required.

Intrahepatic cholestasis of pregnancy (IHCP) is the most common liver disease associated with pregnancy and usually presents in the second and third trimesters. Common symptoms

Table 9.2 Liver diseases unique to pregnancy

Disease	Trimester
Hyperemesis gravidarum	First trimester to 20 weeks
Intrahepatic cholestasis of pregnancy	Second to third trimester
Preeclampsia, eclampsia	After 20 weeks to postpartum
HELLP	After 22 weeks
Acute fatty liver of pregnancy	Third trimester, can continue to postpartum period

include persistent pruritus, usually affecting the palms and soles, and elevated bile acid levels. Bile acids concentrations in IHCP are usually >10 micromol/L with increased cholic acid levels and decreased chenodeoxycholic acid levels. Most complications occur when the bile acid levels exceed 40 micromol/L. AST and ALT can be elevated to >1000 U/L. Maternal outcomes are excellent, but there is a risk of fetal distress, preterm labor, prematurity, and intrauterine death usually in the last month of pregnancy. The treatment is ursodeoxycholic acid at 10–15 mg/kg maternal weight, but IHCP usually resolves with delivery.

Preeclampsia is new-onset hypertension (systolic blood pressure >/= 140 mm Hg or diastolic blood pressure >/=90 mm Hg) and proteinuria (>/=300 mg/24 h) after 20 weeks of gestation. Severe preeclampsia is defined by organ dysfunction including hepatomegaly and hepatocellular injury. Eclampsia occurs when grand mal seizures occur with preeclampsia. Delivery is the only curative treatment.

HELLP syndrome is defined as hemolytic anemia, increased liver enzymes, and low platelets. HELLP usually presents at 28–36 weeks of gestation, but 30% can present in the first week postpartum. The patient presents with thrombocytopenia, elevated AST, ALT, bilirubin, and LDH. Jaundice is only seen in up to 5% of patients. Hypertension and proteinuria are common, seen in up to 80% of patients. Maternal mortality rates are 1–3% in HELLP syndrome. Hepatic complications include hepatic infarction, subcapsular hematomas, and intraparenchymal hemorrhage. Lab values usually begin to normalize 48 h postpartum. If symptoms do not resolve and the patient shows evidence of liver failure, liver transplantation may need to be considered.

Acute fatty liver of pregnancy (AFLP) is rare and can be life-threatening. It is associated with microvesicular fatty infiltration of the liver leading to hepatic failure. AFLP is usually diagnosed around 36 weeks gestation, and prognosis is dependent on the interval between symptoms and termination of the pregnancy. Patients usually present with markedly elevated liver enzymes

Table 9.3 Swansea criteria for the diagnosis of acute fatty liver of pregnancy (AFLP)

Six or more of the following without other causes for these symptoms or signs
Vomiting
Abdominal pain
Polydipsia/polyuria
Encephalopathy
Elevated bilirubin
Hypoglycemia
Elevated urea
Leukocytosis
Ascites or bright liver on ultrasound
Elevated AST/ALT
Elevated ammonia
Renal impairment
Coagulopathy – elevated prothrombin time
Microvesicular steatosis on liver biopsy

and jaundice. Hepatic failure can present with encephalopathy, coagulopathy, hypoglycemia, and organ failure. AFLP can be diagnosed using the Swansea criteria (Table 9.3). Spontaneous recovery does not occur without delivery of the infant. Uncommonly, if hepatic function does not improve after delivery, liver transplant offers the best chance for maternal survival.

Additional Clinical Information and Test Results and Interpretation

Our patient's HAV IgM was negative. Her HBsAg was positive, HBcIgM was negative, HBc total antibody was positive, and HBV DNA was 500,000 IU/mL. Her HCV antibody was negative. Hepatitis E and HSV serologies were not checked given the fact that she was asymptomatic and only had mild elevation of her liver enzymes. She was diagnosed with chronic HBV. The decision was made to start her on tenofovir during the third trimester of pregnancy. The plan was for the baby to also receive hepatitis B immunoglobulin and HBV vaccines at birth.

Conclusions

There are several physiologic changes in the liver which are seen during pregnancy. While albumin may decrease and alkaline phosphatase may increase normally during pregnancy, changes in AST, ALT, or bilirubin should prompt further evaluation. Viral hepatitis, either acute or chronic, should be considered during pregnancy. Effective therapies, especially against hepatitis B, can reduce the risk of transmission to the baby. There are also liver diseases which are unique to pregnancy which must be considered. These can be identified based on clinical signs and symptoms as well as the presenting trimester.

Further Reading

1. AASLD/IDSA recommendations for testing, managing, and treating hepatitis C. www.hcvguidelines.org
2. Brennan PN, Donnelly MC, Simpson KJ. Systematic review: non A-E, seronegative or indeterminate hepatitis; what is this deadly disease? Aliment Pharmacol Ther. 2018;47:1079–91.
3. CDC morbidity and mortality weekly report. www.cdc.gov/mmwr
4. Copel J, El-Sayed Y, Heine RP, Wharton KR. Guidelines for diagnostic imaging during pregnancy and lactations. Obstet Gynecol. 2017;130:e210–6.
5. Ryan J, Heneghan M. Pregnancy and liver. Clinical Liver Disease. 2014;4:51–4.

6. Terrault NA, Bzowej NH, Chang KM, Hwant J, Jonas MM, Murad MH. AASLD guidelines for treatment of chronic hepatitis B. Hepatology. 2016;63:261–83.
7. Tran TT, Ahn J, Reau NS. ACG clinical guidelines: liver disease and pregnancy. Am J Gastroenterol. 2016;111:176–94.

Chapter 10
Asymptomatic, Nonmalignant Liver Masses: A Radiologist's Approach

Raj Mohan Paspulati

Introduction

Asymptomatic liver mass lesions are incidental findings on imaging performed for non-hepatic indications. Advances in radiological imaging and easy availability have led to more frequent use of imaging, resulting in detection of asymptomatic liver lesions. In addition, screening protocols such as CT colonography and cardiac and lung cancer CT screening which include the upper abdomen have resulted in the detection of more incidental liver lesions. These incidental liver lesions have not only created unnecessary concern and apprehension for the patients but also management dilemmas for the clinician. In this chapter, we describe a case of a patient with an incidental liver mass. We briefly discuss the epidemiology and clinical features and focus on the radiologic characteristics of some of the more commonly seen liver benign lesions.

R. M. Paspulati
Digestive Health Institute, Head of GI and GYN Radiology, Division of Abdominal Imaging, Department of Radiology, University Hospitals, Case Western Reserve University, Cleveland, OH, USA
e-mail: Raj.Paspulati@UHhospitals.org

© Springer Nature Switzerland AG 2019
S. M. Cohen, P. Davitkov (eds.), *Liver Disease*,
https://doi.org/10.1007/978-3-319-98506-0_10

Clinical Case Scenario

A 34-year-old female is referred by her primary care physician for an incidentally discovered liver mass. She has had frequent urinary tract infections. As part of that evaluation, she underwent a renal ultrasound (US) that demonstrates normal kidneys and also notes a 4 cm lesion in the right lobe of the liver. She takes no medications other than a multivitamin. She is on no oral contraceptive pills. She has no past history of known liver disease, liver masses, or malignancy. She does not ever recall getting prior imaging studies of her liver. There is no known family history of liver disease or malignancy. Her physical examination is completely unremarkable. Laboratory data including CBC and comprehensive panel are completely normal.

Questions

1. What are the various imaging modalities used for characterizing liver masses?
2. What are some of the common nonmalignant liver masses, and what are the epidemiology and features of these lesions?
3. What are the radiologic features of these lesions?

Discussion

Question 1. What are the various imaging modalities used for characterizing liver masses?

With improvements in imaging modalities and more frequent use of such studies, incidental liver lesions are being seen more commonly. Studies have shown that incidental liver lesions are detected in about 30% of individuals aged 40 years and above. However, the percentage of these incidental liver lesions which are clinically significant and require management is very low. Nearly 50% of these are considered completely benign on initial imaging, and the other 50% fall into the category of indeterminate or worrisome lesions that need further imaging for definitive characterization.

Because of its low cost, lack of ionizing radiation, and wide availability, US is the most common initial imaging study which identifies an incidental liver lesion. Generally, follow-up imaging to better characterize and identify lesions is done with contrast-enhanced MRI or CT. Contrast-enhanced imaging studies examine a variety of timed sequences including pre-contrast phase, early arterial contrast phase, later venous contrast phase, and delayed phases. Multiphase contrast MRI has become the preferred imaging modality at most medical centers. A triple-phase, contrast-enhanced CT and contrast-enhanced US are alternative imaging methods in patients who cannot undergo an MRI due to claustrophobia or other contraindications for MRI. Nuclear medicine studies are now rarely used in the evaluation of liver lesions. Imaging features of some of the common incidentally detected asymptomatic hepatic mass lesions are illustrated in this chapter.

Question 2. What are some of the common nonmalignant liver masses, and what are the epidemiology and features of these lesions?

Hepatic hemangiomas are the most common benign hepatic masses discovered incidentally on routine imaging, with an incidence of 0.4–20% in the general population. They have a slightly higher prevalence in females. Hepatic hemangiomas are composed of sinusoidal spaces lined by endothelial cells and intervening fibrous septa. They generally range in size from a few millimeters to 20 centimeters. They are usually solitary but can be multiple in about 10% of patients. Hemangiomas over 5 cm in size are termed "giant hemangiomas." Sclerosing hemangiomas have extensive fibrosis with near-complete obliteration of the sinusoidal vascular spaces. Hence, these hemangiomas do not have the characteristic imaging features of a typical hemangioma.

Focal nodular hyperplasia (FNH) is the second most common benign hepatic lesion detected incidentally on routine abdominal imaging. It is not a true tumor and is due to focal hyperplasia of normal hepatic parenchyma due to increased arterial flow from an occult developmental arterial malformation. It has a reported prevalence of 0.9% and has an approximately eight times higher incidence in females than males. Multiple FNH are seen in 20% and can be associated with hemangiomas. FNH can vary in size from a few mm to 10 cm and can present as an exophytic mass from the liver surface. Gross pathology of a typical FNH consists of a well-demarcated, unencapsulated mass and central stellate scar with radiating septa separating nodules of hepatic parenchyma. Histopathology reveals normal hepatocytes within the nodular hyperplastic parenchyma separated by fibrous septa which can be complete or incomplete. The central stellate scar has interstitial fibrosis, proliferating ductules without a large draining duct, and tortuous arteries with thick walls and veins.

Hepatocellular adenomas are benign tumors commonly seen in women using oral contraceptives for over 2 years. Other risk factors include prolonged use of anabolic steroids and type 1 glycogen storage disease. Type 1 glycogen storage disease can also be associated with multiple hepatic adenomas. Liver adenomatosis is a distinct entity presenting with multiple hepatic adenomas (>10) in patients without any predisposing risk factors. Hepatic adenomas can vary in size from 1 cm to >15 cm. Traditionally, all hepatic adenomas were managed by surgical excision due to the increased risk of spontaneous hemorrhage and potential risk of malignant transformation into hepatocellular carcinoma (HCC). However, recent studies have shown that adenomas are a spectrum of disease with several subtypes having different genetic and pathological abnormalities. Not all of them are at increased risk of hemorrhage or malignant transformation and need not be subjected to surgical excision. Hepatic adenomas are currently classified into three subtypes based on genetic and histopathologic features. The three subtypes are (1) inflammatory adenomas; (2) hepatocyte nuclear factor 1 alpha (HNF-1α)-mutated adenomas; and (3) β-catenin-mutated adenomas. Hepatic adenomas without any associated genetic abnormalities are categorized as "unclassified." Of the three subtypes, inflammatory and HNF-1α-mutated adenomas have distinct histopathologic and imaging findings. MR imaging can be useful in identifying these subtypes without biopsy (see imaging characteristics below). Inflammatory adenomas are the most common subtype (40–50% of all adenomas). They are most commonly seen in young, obese women with oral contraceptive use. This subtype has the highest risk of hemorrhage. HNF-1α-mutated adenomas are the second most common subtype (30–35%). They can be seen in maturity-onset diabetes of the young (MODY) type 3 and familial hepatic adenomatosis. The β-catenin subtypes represent 10–15% of adenomas. They are more common in men and associated with the use of anabolic steroids, glycogen storage disease, and familial adenomatous polyposis. This subtype has the highest risk of malignancy. Histopathology of adenomas reveals plates of normal hepatocytes separated by sinusoids with no bile ductules, a key histologic finding differentiating them from an FNH. The Kupffer cells are also either reduced in number or function, another feature useful in differentiating from an FNH.

Hepatic cysts are commonly identified incidental asymptomatic mass lesions detected on routine imaging. Solitary unilocular simple cysts without associated congenital polycystic hepatic and/or renal disease are seen in 2.5–18% of the general population. They can vary in size from <1 cm to very large cysts essentially replacing the entire liver lobes. Large cysts can be symptomatic due to significant mass effect. Hemorrhage within the cysts as well as degenerative changes within the cyst due to desquamation, septation, and calcification can make them appear complex. These complex cysts can be mistaken for hydatid cysts or biliary cystadenomas. Histopathology of a simple cyst shows a uniformly thin collagenous wall lined by a flat or cuboidal biliary-type epithelium.

In addition to the above masses which are true lesions, there are a number of pseudo-lesions or pseudotumors which may be commonly reported by the radiologist. While benign or essentially artefactual, these can be of concern to the patient and provider. We will briefly mention focal fatty infiltration, focal fatty sparing, and hepatic vascular shunts and discuss their radiologic findings below. Fatty liver disease is the most common liver in the USA. While imaging usually reveals diffuse fatty changes, there can be patients who have only focal areas of fatty change (focal fatty infiltration) or focal areas of fatty sparing (essentially areas of normal liver in a background of an otherwise fatty liver). Hepatic vascular shunts are just areas of enhanced blood flow identified on imaging studies. They are not of clinical significance but can mimic other tumors.

Additional Clinical Information

The patient is seen in the liver clinic. She gets an alpha-fetoprotein level which is normal. She then gets an MRI which reveals a 4 cm lesion in the right lobe of the liver. The lesion is hyperintense with a non-enhancing central scar. Her case is reviewed at the weekly tumor board conference.

Question 3. What are the radiologic features of these lesions?

Typical or Classic Hemangiomas

The imaging features of a classic hemangioma depend upon the size of the sinusoidal spaces and the relative composition of the fibrous stroma. Hemangiomas up to 3 cm have classic imaging features. Larger hemangiomas have more fibrous stroma and can have varying degree of central thrombosis and rarely calcification resulting in atypical imaging features.

Ultrasound

A typical hemangioma on US is seen as a well-defined echogenic lesion with sharp margins and has posterior acoustic enhancement. Doppler US shows no arterial or venous flow within the echogenic mass (see Fig. 10.1). In a steatotic liver, hemangioma

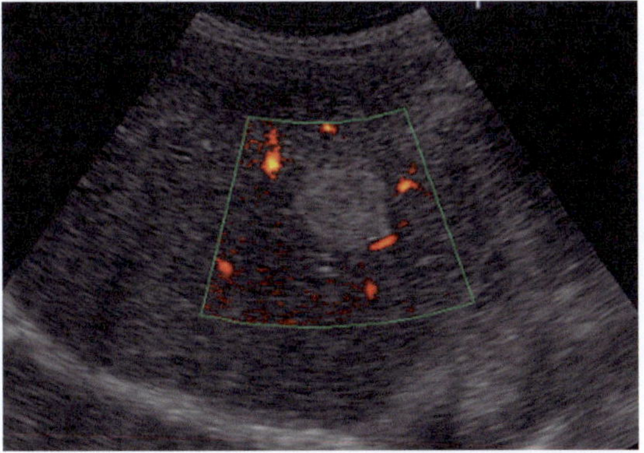

Fig. 10.1 Ultrasonography of hemangioma. A well-defined echogenic lesion in the right hepatic lobe without vascular flow on color Doppler imaging

can be hypoechoic due to the echogenic surrounding hepatic parenchyma and can be mistaken for primary or secondary hepatic malignancy. Contrast-enhanced ultrasonography (CEUS) following IV administration of a microbubble US contrast agent can demonstrate slow sinusoidal flow within a hemangioma, not seen with Doppler US. On CEUS, typical hemangiomas demonstrate initial peripheral nodular enhancement with gradual centripetal filling.

CT

A typical hemangioma has low attenuation on non-enhanced CT with attenuation similar to hepatic vasculature. On contrast-enhanced CT, there is an initial peripheral nodular, interrupted pattern of enhancement in the arterial dominant phase with gradual central filling in the portal venous and delayed images. The enhancement persists on delayed-phase images due to contrast retention within the sinusoids (see Fig. 10.2a, b).

MRI

A typical hemangioma on MRI has high signal intensity on T2-weighted images similar to a fluid-filled cyst ("light-bulb sign," see Fig. 10.3a) and has low signal intensity on non-enhanced T1-weighted images (see Fig. 10.3b). The imaging features are similar to contrast CT on serial post-gadolinium-enhanced T1-weighted images. There is initial peripheral nodular, interrupted enhancement with gradual centripetal filling and retention of contrast on delayed images (see Fig. 10.3c).

Nuclear Medicine Scans

Technetium-labeled RBC scintigraphy has been completely replaced by MRI for definitive imaging of a suspected hemangioma. With this scan, there is no uptake in the initial dynamic

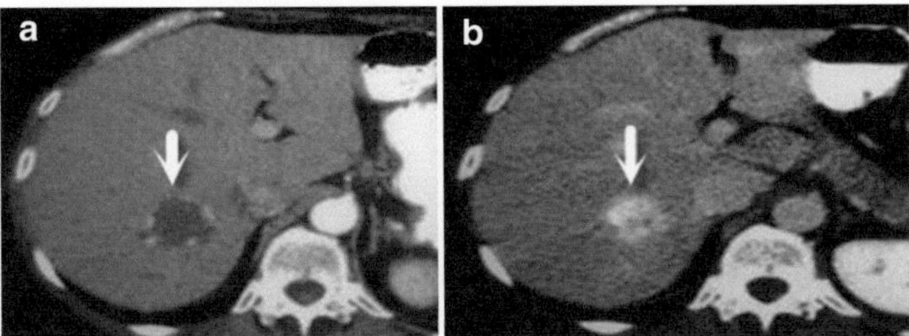

Fig. 10.2 Contrast-enhanced CT of hemangioma. Contrast-enhanced CT images of the liver in early arterial dominant phase (**a**) and delayed phase (**b**) demonstrate initial peripheral, interrupted nodular enhancement with complete filling on delayed images

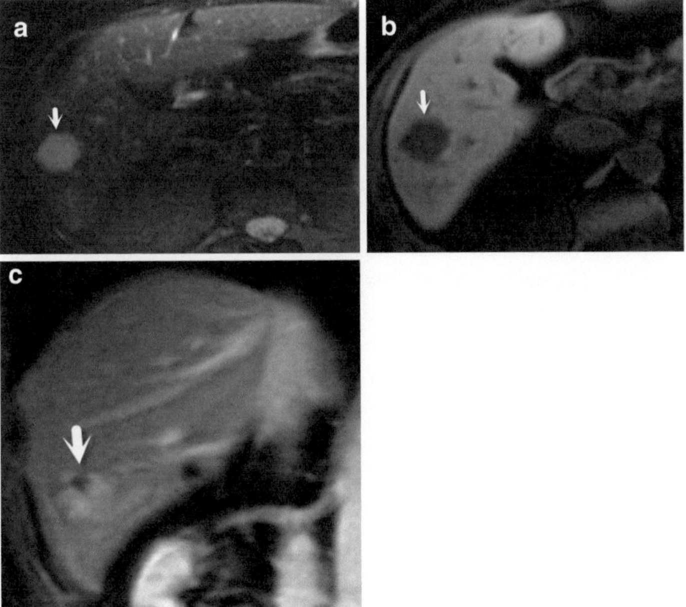

Fig. 10.3 MRI of a classic hemangioma. A well-defined right hepatic lobe mass, hyperintense of fluid signal intensity on T2-weighted image (**a**), hypointense on T1-weighted image (**b**) with progressive centripetal enhancement on dynamic post gadolinium T1-weighted images (**c**)

imaging with increased uptake on delayed images and retention on delayed images at 30–60 min.

Atypical Hemangiomas

Up to 40% of hepatic hemangiomas can have atypical imaging features due to varying degrees of hemorrhagic necrosis, thrombosis, cystic change, fibrosis, and myxomatous change. This is usually seen with hemangiomas measuring 4 cm and larger.

On US, these atypical hemangiomas are not homogeneously hyperechoic and are partially hypoechoic due to central degenerative changes. Most of them retain a peripheral echogenic rim and are avascular on color Doppler US. Giant hemangiomas, on MR imaging, have linear or cleft-like hyperintense foci due to cystic degeneration or liquefaction and hypointense septa due to central scar on T2-weighted images. The enhancement pattern is similar to CT with incomplete central filling and no enhancement of the central fibrous septa and clefts (see Fig. 10.4a–c).

Small hemangiomas measuring less than 1 cm can demonstrate complete enhancement in the initial arterial dominant phase of the CT and MRI due to the small sinusoids filling in rapidly. These are called "flash-filling hemangiomas" and can have focal, transient hepatic parenchymal enhancement surrounding the hemangioma due to arterio-portal shunting. They can be mistaken for HCC or hypervascular metastases, but, unlike malignant lesions, they do not have venous phase washout and retain contrast on delayed images.

Sclerosing hemangiomas have extensive fibrosis with near-complete obliteration of the sinusoidal vascular spaces. Hence, these hemangiomas do not have the characteristic imaging features of a typical hemangioma. On CT, these hemangiomas have heterogeneous nodular areas of enhancement on delayed images or no significant enhancement. On MRI, they have low signal intensity on T2-weighted images representing areas of fibrosis and hyaline change and persistent delayed enhancement of these T2-hypointense foci. Peripheral sclerosing hemangiomas

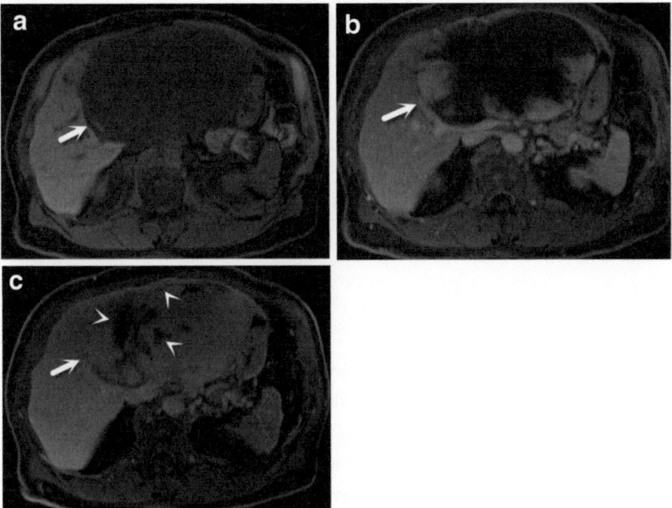

Fig. 10.4 Giant hemangioma with atypical features. T1-weighted MR image (**a**) shows a large hypointense mass. On dynamic post-gadolinium T1-weighted images (**b**), there is initial peripheral nodular enhancement with more progressive centripetal enhancement, and the delayed image (**c**) shows complete enhancement with central non-enhancing foci of cystic change and fibrosis (arrow heads)

can cause capsular retraction. Some of these are difficult to differentiate from cholangiocarcinoma or metastases and, in the right clinical setting, may need biopsy and histopathology confirmation.

Typical Focal Nodular Hyperplasia (FNH)

Ultrasound

Sonographic findings of FNH may be subtle. Small FNH may not be visualized on US. Larger FNH can be isoechoic, hypoechoic, or slightly hyperechoic to normal hepatic parenchyma. A hyperechoic central scar with radiating septa may be identified in large FNH. A peripheral hypoechoic halo can be seen with some FNH due to compressed surrounding hepatic parenchyma. Doppler US may demonstrate radiating arterial flow from the central scar to the periphery in a spoke–wheel pattern. Contrast-enhanced US will demonstrate diffusely increased echogenicity in the arterial phase and may demonstrate a central feeding artery with spoke–wheel pattern to the periphery.

CT

The characteristic enhancing features of FNH are better evaluated on multiphase contrast-enhanced CT imaging. FNH is isoattenuating or hypoattenuating to the surrounding liver on unenhanced images. In the arterial phase, there is homogeneous hyperenhancement of the lesion except for the central scar. In the portal and delayed venous phases, it is isoattenuating to the surrounding hepatic parenchyma, and the central scar will be hyperintense due to delayed enhancement.

MRI

On MRI, a typical FNH is isointense or minimally hyperintense relative to the surrounding hepatic parenchyma on T2-weighted images and isointense or hypointense on unenhanced T1-weighted images. The central scar is hyperintense on T2-weighted images. On dynamic contrast-enhanced images, it shows homogeneous intense enhancement except for the central scar in the arterial dominant phase and becomes isointense in the portal and delayed venous phases with delayed enhancement of the central scar (see Fig. 10.5).

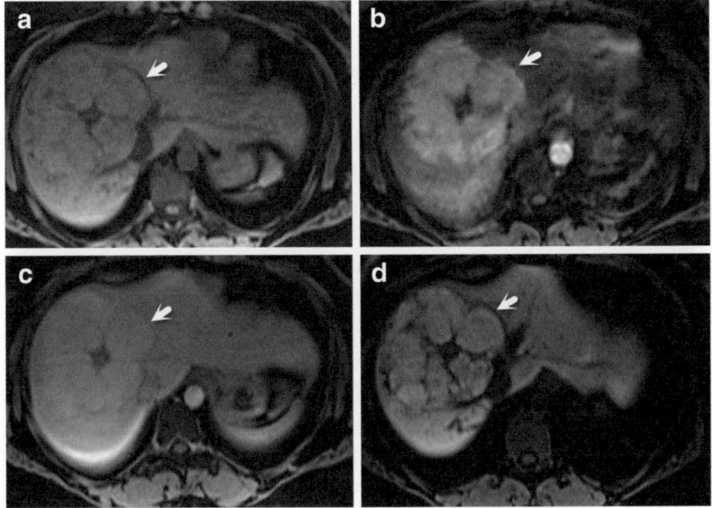

Fig. 10.5 Typical FNH on MRI. Pre-contrast (**a**) and post-contrast T1-weighted images in arterial (**b**), portal venous (**c**), and delayed hepatobiliary (**d**) phases show characteristic intense enhancement with a non-enhancing scar in the arterial phase, remaining minimally hyperintense in the portal venous phase and hyperintense to the hepatic parenchyma in the hepatobiliary phase with a central hypointense scar (arrow head)

Nuclear Medicine Scans

On technetium-99m sulfur colloid scan, FNH may demonstrate similar or increased uptake compared to normal liver parenchyma in approximately 60% of patients due to the presence of sufficient numbers of functioning Kupffer cells. Due to the higher sensitivity and specificity of MRI, scintigraphy is no longer a preferred imaging modality for the diagnosis of FNH.

Atypical FNH

Small FNH may appear as transient enhancing lesions in the arterial phase and become isointense and undetectable in the portal venous phase of contrast-enhanced CT. They do not have the central scar and can be mistaken for vascular shunts.

Approximately 20% of FNH may not have typical imaging features on a dynamic contrast-enhanced MRI. The FNH can be hypointense on T2-weighted images without a central hyperintense scar. The central scar may be hypointense and may not show typical delayed enhancement. It may have heterogeneous signal intensity on T2-weighted images and may not show typical homogenous enhancement in the arterial phase. In an asymptomatic young patient, atypical FNH may be difficult to differentiate from an adenoma or HCC. MR imaging with gadolinium-based contrast or gadoxetic acid-based contrast (Eovist®) can be useful in this situation. The sensitivity and specificity for differentiation of FNH and adenoma with hepatobiliary contrast MRI are 96–100%.

Hepatocellular Adenomas

As noted above, hepatocellular adenomas are classified into three main subtypes: (1) inflammatory adenomas, (2) hepatocyte nuclear factor 1 alpha (HNF-1α)-mutated adenomas, and (3) β-catenin-mutated adenomas. Hepatic adenomas without any associated genetic abnormalities are considered unclassified.

Hepatocellular adenomas have to be differentiated from other hypervascular hepatic lesions in young individuals without underlying chronic liver disease and cirrhosis. These include FNH, fibrolamellar HCC, and hypervascular metastases.

Inflammatory Hepatocellular Adenomas

Ultrasound

Imaging features on US are nonspecific. They can be hypoechoic or heterogeneous depending on the degree of sinusoidal dilation and the presence of intrinsic hemorrhage (see Fig. 10.6). Color Doppler US may show a variable degree of arterial and venous flow.

CT

On non-enhanced CT, they may be heterogeneous in attenuation due to foci of hyperattenuation secondary to hemorrhage. On contrast-enhanced CT, they enhance in the arterial phase with retention of contrast on delayed venous phase due to pooling of contrast in the sinusoidal spaces similar to a hemangioma.

MRI

MR imaging features are characteristic and have high sensitivity (85%) and specificity (87%) in the diagnosis of inflammatory adenomas (see Fig. 10.6b–e). They are hyperintense on T2-weighted images and hypointense on pre-gadolinium T1-weighted images and will have foci of high T1 signal intensity in the presence of hemorrhage. Minimal or no signal drop on chemical shift T1-weighted images indicates no significant intralesion lipid. Enhancing features on post-gadolinium T1 images are similar to contrast-enhanced CT with intense enhancement in the arterial phase with persistent enhancement on delayed images without washout. With gadoxetic acid-based contrast, they will be hypointense on delayed

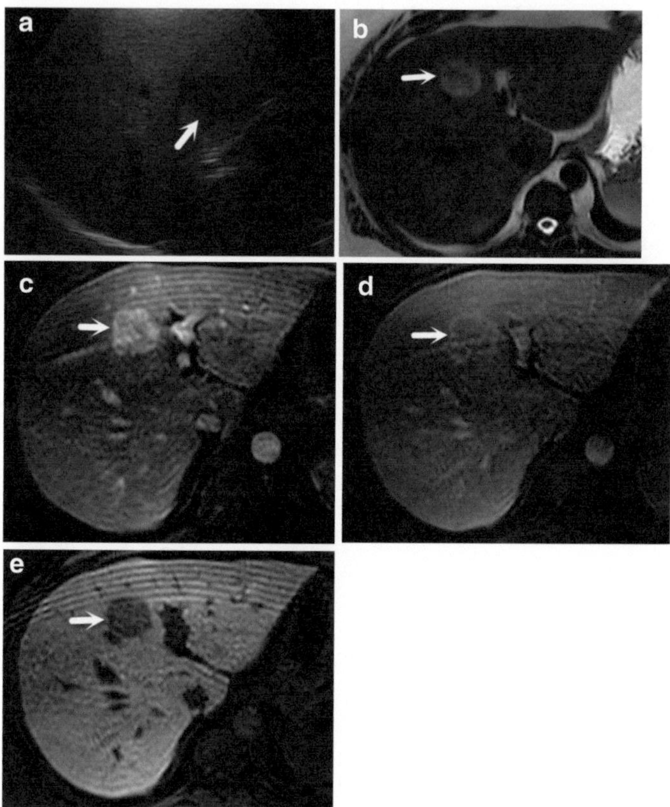

Fig. 10.6 Inflammatory adenoma. Ultrasound images depict a hypoechoic mass in the right hepatic lobe without vascular flow (**a**). MRI shows diffuse hyperintense signal intensity of the mass on T2-weighted image (**b**) and intense enhancement in the arterial phase (**c**), mild persistent enhancement in the delayed phase (**d**), and hypointense relative to the background hepatic parenchyma in the hepatobiliary phase image (**e**)

hepatobiliary phase images. Steatosis of the background hepatic parenchyma is more commonly associated with this subtype. Spontaneous hemorrhage can be the initial presentation of inflammatory adenomas. The presence of hemorrhage at the acute presentation may mask the typical imaging features. Hemorrhage is seen as hyperattenuating foci on unenhanced T1-weighted MR images.

HNF-1α-Mutated Hepatocellular Adenomas

Ultrasound/CT

These adenomas can be hyperechoic on US and show variable degrees of low attenuation on contrast-enhanced CT due to intralesion lipid content (see Fig. 10.7a).

MRI

On MR imaging, these lesions show intrinsic variable degree of drop in signal intensity on out-of-phase T1 chemical shift images due to intracellular lipid (see Fig. 10.7b). They are either isointense or minimally hyperintense on T2-weighted images. There is mild to moderate enhancement in the arterial phase images with no persistent enhancement on delayed-phase images. Steatosis of the background hepatic parenchyma is seen on T1 out-of-phase chemical shift images. Chemical shift MR imaging has higher sensitivity (86%) and specificity (100%) in the detection of intralesion lipid characteristics of this subtype of hepatic adenoma (see Fig. 10.7c).

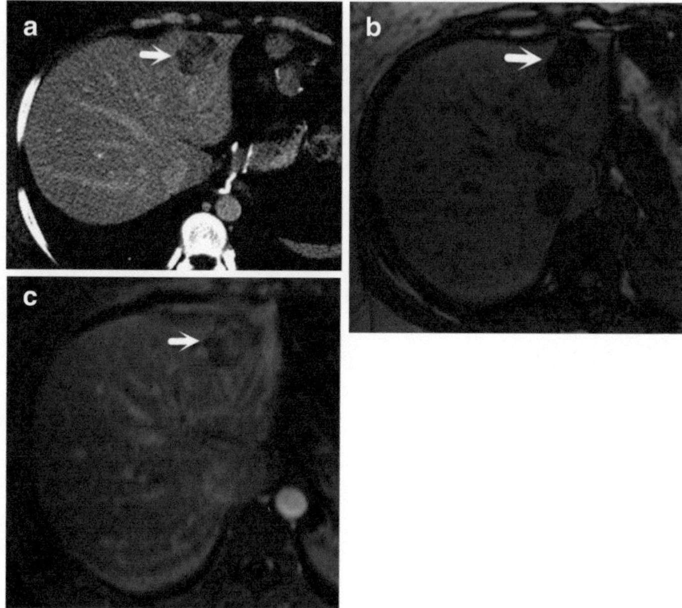

Fig. 10.7 HNF-1α-mutated hepatocellular adenoma. Axial contrast-enhanced CT image in portal venous phase (**a**) shows a heterogeneously enhancing mass with low-attenuation foci. MR imaging shows intrinsic lipid within the mass by drop in signal intensity on out-of-phase T1-weighted image (**b**). Heterogeneous enhancement of the mass on delayed dynamic post-gadolinium images is demonstrated (**c**)

β-Catenin-Mutated Hepatocellular Adenomas

Imaging features of this subtype are nonspecific and can mimic features of HCC.

MRI

They may be homogeneously or heterogeneously hyperintense on T1-weighted images depending upon the presence of hemorrhage and necrosis. They show intense enhancement in the arterial dominant phase and may or may not show persistent enhancement in the portal and delayed-phase images. Biopsy and histopathology may be necessary to differentiate from HCC.

Simple Hepatic Cysts

Ultrasound

A simple hepatic cyst is seen as anechoic mass with through transmission, surrounded by a thin wall and no internal septations or minimal thin septations.

CT

Contrast-enhanced CT shows a well-defined mass of fluid attenuation with a thin enhancing wall (see Fig. 10.8a).

MRI

MRI shows a well-defined T2 hyperintense mass with a hypointense thin wall. Cyst contents are hypointense on T1-weighted images with a thin enhancing wall (see Fig. 10.8b, c).

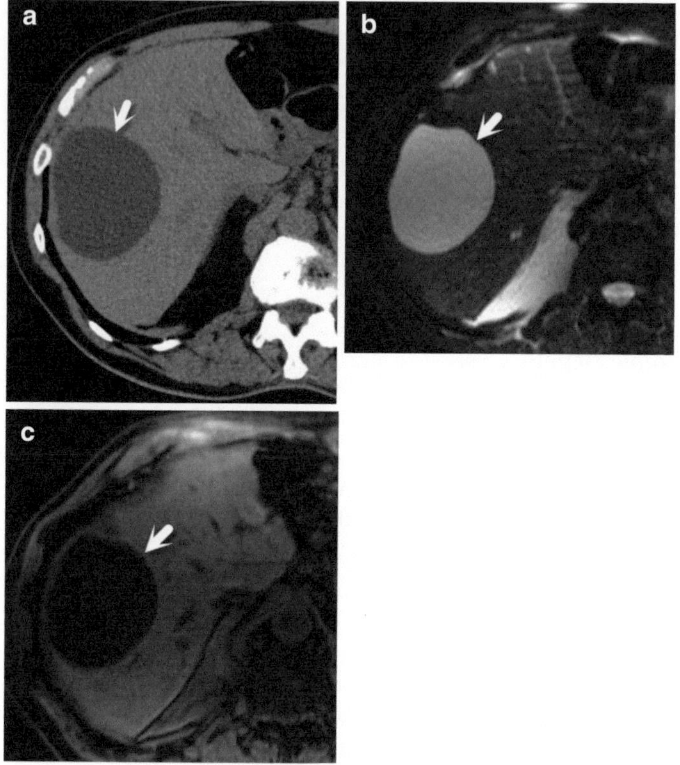

Fig. 10.8 Simple hepatic cyst. Unenhanced CT image (**a**) shows a large well-defined mass (arrow) of fluid attenuation. On MRI, the mass is intensely hyperintense on a T2-weighted image (**b**) and hypointense on a T1-weighted image (**c**)

Complex Hepatic Cysts

Ultrasound/CT/MRI

Complex cysts due to hemorrhage or desquamation may show thin or thick non-enhancing septations, thickened walls, calcification from prior hemorrhage, or even evidence of active hemorrhage (see Fig. 10.9). These complex cysts have to be

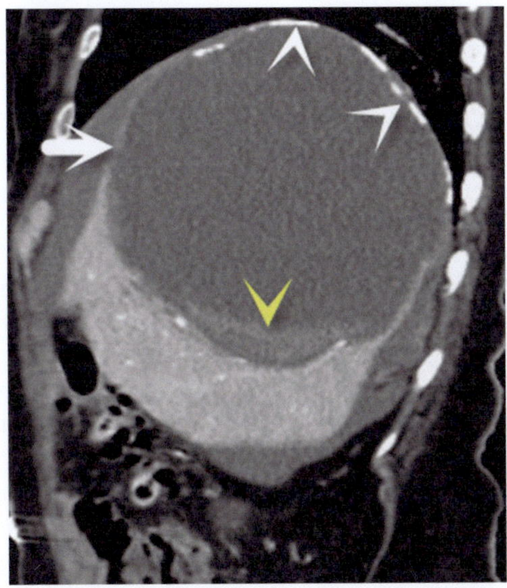

Fig. 10.9 Complex hemorrhagic cyst. Sagittal contrast-enhanced CT image shows a large well-defined mass in the right lobe of fluid attenuation with a thick calcified wall (white arrow heads) and dependent layering hyperdensity (yellow arrow head) indicating hemorrhage. No enhancing mural nodules are seen

differentiated from biliary cystadenomas or echinococcal (hydatid) cysts in endemic areas. Cystadenomas usually have thick, enhancing septations and mural nodularity. Some complex simple hepatic cysts cannot be differentiated from cystadenomas and may need cyst fluid aspiration or excision for a definitive diagnosis.

Focal Fatty Infiltration

Focal fatty infiltration on US and CT can occasionally have a nodular appearance mimicking a mass lesion. MRI with T1 imaging can identify these as focal areas of steatosis.

Focal Fatty Sparing

Focal fatty sparing in an otherwise steatotic liver can have a mass-like appearance on US and CT. On US, focal fatty sparing is hypoechoic against a background of echogenic fatty liver. On contrast-enhanced CT, it is hyperattenuating compared to the low-attenuation steatotic hepatic parenchyma. Typical fatty sparing is wedge-shaped with a characteristic location in segments 4 and 5, adjacent to gallbladder fossa. Fatty sparring can also be nodular and in atypical locations and can mimic a neoplastic mass lesion. MRI with T1 chemical shift imaging, diffusion-weighted imaging, and dynamic post-gadolinium imaging is useful in differentiating them from true tumors.

Hepatic Vascular Shunts

Hepatic vascular shunts are seen as focal enhancing areas within the liver on US or a routine single-phase contrast-enhanced study and can mimic an enhancing liver mass such as hemangioma, FNH, or a hypervascular malignancy. Follow-up with either a triple-phase CT or MRI can identify them as benign vascular shunts of no clinical significance, with no need for further evaluation. The shunts can be either arterio-portal or portosystemic between a peripheral branch of the portal vein and the hepatic vein. The arterio-portal shunts are seen as peripheral wedge-shaped foci of transient parenchymal enhancement, becoming isointense with the normal enhancing parenchyma in portal and delayed venous phases. On MRI, there is no associated abnormal signal intensity in the T2-weighted images and unenhanced T1-weighted images with similar enhancing features to CT on post-contrast images. The arterio-portal shunts can be seen in the normal liver but are more commonly seen in cirrhotic livers and can be a manifestation of compromised portal venous flow secondary to more proximal portal vein thrombosis or compression. The arterio-portal shunts secondary to compromised portal venous flow are much larger and geographic, located in the area of compromised portal venous flow.

Patient Clinical Course

The patient is reviewed at the tumor board. Based on the radiologic findings, the lesion is felt to be a classic focal nodular hyperplasia. This is a benign lesion. In this asymptomatic patient, no further evaluation or follow-up is deemed necessary.

Conclusions

Incidental asymptomatic liver mass lesions are not uncommon due to more frequent use of imaging studies. Most of these incidental hepatic mass lesions are benign and do not need further management or follow up. However, some need more advanced imaging by multiphase MRI or CT for further characterization.

Selected References

1. Nguyen XV, Davies L, Eastwood JD, Hoang JK. Extrapulmonary findings and malignancies in participants screened with chest CT in the National Lung Screening Trial. J Am Coll Radiol. 2017;14(3):324–30.
2. Kaltenbach TE, Engler P, Kratzer W, Oeztuerk S, Seufferlein T, Haenle MM, Graeter T. Prevalence of benign focal liver lesions: ultrasound investigation of 45,319 hospital patients. Abdom Radiol. 2016;41(1):25–32.
3. Semelka RC, Sofka CM. Hepatic hemangiomas. Magn Reson Imaging N Am. 1997;5:241–53.
4. Golli M, Mathieu D, Anglade MC, Cherqui D, Vasile N, Rahmouni A. Focal nodular hyperplasia of the liver: value of color Doppler US in association with MR imaging. Radiology. 1993;187(1):113–7.
5. Grazioli L, Morana G, Kirchin MA, Schneider G. Accurate differentiation of focal nodular hyperplasia from hepatic adenoma at gadobenate dimeglumine–enhanced MR imaging: prospective study. Radiology. 2005;236(1):166–77.
6. Zucman-Rossi J, Jeannot E, Nhieu JT, Scoazec JY, Guettier C, Rebouissou S, Bacq Y, Leteurtre E, Paradis V, Michalak S, Wendum D, Chiche L, Fabre M, Mellottee L, Laurent C, Partensky C, Castaing D, Zafrani ES, Laurent-Puig P, Balabaud C, Bioulac-Sage P. Genotype-phenotype correlation in hepatocellular adenoma: new classification and relationship with HCC. Hepatology. 2006;43(3):515–24.
7. Bioulac-Sage P, Balabaud C, Zucman-Rossi J. Subtype classification of hepatocellular adenoma. Dig Surg. 2010;27(1):39–45.
8. Laumonier H, Bioulac-Sage P, Laurent C, Zucman-Rossi J, Balabaud C, Trillaud H. Hepatocellular adenomas: magnetic resonance imaging features as a function of molecular pathological classification. Hepatology. 2008;48(3):808–18.
9. Mavilia MG, Pakala T, Molina M, Wu GY. Differentiating cystic liver lesions: a review of imaging modalities, diagnosis and management. J Clin Transl Hepatol. 2018;6(2):208–16.
10. Lantinga MA, Gevers TJG, Drenth JPH. Evaluation of hepatic cystic lesions. World J Gastroenterol. 2013;19(23):3543–54.
11. Gore RM, et al. Management of incidental liver lesions on CT: a white paper of the ACR incidental findings committee. J Am Coll Radiol. 2017;14(11):1429–37.

Chapter 11
Hepatocellular Carcinoma

Daniel B. Karb and Seth N. Sclair

Introduction

Hepatocellular carcinoma (HCC) is the most common primary cancer of the liver. It generally arises in patients with underlying cirrhosis. Screening and surveillance can be used to identify HCC. Many treatment modalities exist for HCC. In this chapter, we describe a case of a cirrhotic patient found to have HCC. We discuss screening strategies, diagnostic criteria, and treatment options for HCC.

Clinical Case Scenario

A 63-year-old African American male is referred to a liver transplant center for a liver mass. He has a history of alcoholic cirrhosis. He underwent a transjugular intrahepatic portosystemic

D. B. Karb
University Hospitals, Cleveland, OH, USA

S. N. Sclair (✉)
Division of Gastroenterology and Liver Disease, University Hospitals
Cleveland Medical Center, Case Western Reserve University School
of Medicine, Cleveland, OH, USA
e-mail: seth.sclair@uhhospitals.org

© Springer Nature Switzerland AG 2019
S. M. Cohen, P. Davitkov (eds.), *Liver Disease*,
https://doi.org/10.1007/978-3-319-98506-0_11

shunt (TIPS) 5 years previously for severe variceal bleeding. After the TIPS, he stopped all alcohol use and has been clinically stable and well compensated. He has been undergoing routine liver cancer screening with ultrasound and alfa fetoprotein (AFP) testing every 6 months. He did however miss his last cycle of screening and has not had an ultrasound (US) in 1 year. He saw his gastroenterologist who ordered full liver labs as well as an US and AFP. His liver enzymes were significant for an albumin of 3.1 gm/dL, alkaline phosphatase of 160 U/L, and bilirubin of 2.3 mg/dL. His renal panel and INR were normal. His CBC was only significant for a platelet count of 136. His AFP was elevated at 836 ng/mL. The US revealed a 5 cm mass in the hepatic dome.

Questions

1. Should patients with cirrhosis be screened for HCC? What are the current screening and surveillance guidelines for HCC?
2. Once a suspicious lesion is identified on US, what is the next step?
3. How likely is this lesion to be HCC? What are the diagnostic criteria of HCC? Does the patient require a biopsy?
4. How is HCC staged? What is our patient's stage?
5. How should HCC treatment decisions ideally be made?
6. What are the treatment options for this lesion?

Discussion

Question 1. Should patients with cirrhosis be screened for HCC? What are the current screening and surveillance guidelines for HCC?

HCC screening in this patient was appropriate. Patients with cirrhosis are at high risk of developing HCC, with a rate of approximately 3–8% per year, depending on the etiology of cirrhosis.

All patients with cirrhosis, regardless of cause, should at least be considered for screening, and most should actually be screened. Pooled evidence from a systematic review of HCC suggests a mortality benefit in cirrhosis patients who were screened for HCC, which is likely due to early detection and treatment when compared with those patients not screened. Despite clinical practice guidelines and data to support screening, studies have repeatedly demonstrated that HCC screening is underutilized.

Because of the mortality benefit of screening, the American Association for the Study of Liver Diseases (AASLD) strongly recommends screening all adults with cirrhosis, except those with Child's class C cirrhosis who are not eligible for liver transplantation (given the low anticipated survival for these patients). Screening by US at 6-month intervals is the optimal screening modality.

AFP is a glycoprotein that is often elevated in patients with HCC. The addition of AFP to ultrasound screening regimens appears to moderately enhance early HCC detection without a statistically significant effect on mortality. In addition to screening, AFP levels are used in staging, in transplant evaluation, to follow response to treatment, and to detect recurrence of disease. Note that AFP levels do not correlate with other features of HCC, such as size, stage, or prognosis.

Question 2. Once a suspicious lesion is identified on US, what is the next step?

Lesions that are suspicious for HCC and > 1 cm in diameter should undergo further imaging with either multiphasic CT or MRI. Unlike most other malignancies, the diagnosis of HCC can be established noninvasively by imaging studies. In addition to diagnosis, this imaging is also used for tumor staging.

There is no consensus about which imaging modality to use (MRI or CT), as long as multiphasic studies are obtained. Depending on the imaging modality of choice, the contrast agent, and the size and location of the lesion, pooled sensitivity estimates range from 60% to 90% with specificity of 80–90%. Multiphasic MRI may be marginally more sensitive than multiphasic CT (especially for smaller lesions). Both modalities require the use of intravenous contrast agents, and caution must be used in patients with acute or chronic kidney disease.

Question 3. How likely is this lesion to be HCC? What are the diagnostic criteria of HCC? Does the patient require a biopsy?

The American College of Radiology (ACR) has endorsed the Liver Imaging Reporting and Data System (LI-RADS) classification system for estimating the likelihood of HCC in at-risk patients. The LI-RADS algorithm assigns each lesion a likelihood of HCC based on several primary features of the lesion including size, arterial phase enhancement, washout hypoenhancement, enhancing capsule, and threshold growth. Using these criteria, each lesion is classified into one of five major categories: LR-1 (definitely benign), LR-2 (probably benign), LR-3 (intermediate probability of malignancy), LR-4 (probably HCC), and LR-5 (definitely HCC).

LR-5 lesions are considered definitely HCC and do not require a biopsy for diagnosis. Exceptions might be made when there is a concern for a mixed tumor such as HCC and cholangiocarcinoma which is treated differently than HCC alone.

Prior versions of HCC clinical practice guidelines recommended biopsy for all indeterminate lesions initially detected by surveillance ultrasound (e.g., LR-3 lesion), but the AASLD no longer recommends routine biopsy for these lesions. The evidence suggests that a substantial percentage of indeterminate, small lesions (<2 cm) are nonmalignant, and biopsy at the time of initial discovery would result in a large number of unnecessary procedures. However, these lesions do require further follow-up. Options include follow-up imaging or imaging with an alternative modality or contrast agent. Biopsy may be warranted in selected cases of indeterminate imaging.

A triple-phase MRI is performed and reveals a 7.0×5.2 cm mass in segment 7. The radiologist reports that this is an LR-5 lesion, diagnostic for HCC. No biopsy was deemed necessary to make the diagnosis. Chest CT reveals no evidence of metastatic disease.

Question 4. How is HCC staged? What is our patient's stage?

Multiple HCC staging and prognostic systems exist, none of which has been universally adopted. For the purposes of this chapter, we will review only the Barcelona Clinic Liver Cancer (BCLC) staging system, which is a widely used staging algorithm that includes treatment recommendations (see Table 11.1).

Table 11.1 Barcelona Clinic Liver Cancer (BCLC) staging system

BCLC stage	Characterization	Tumor characteristics	Treatment recommendations
0	Very early stage	Single nodule <2 cm	Curative Resection or transplant
A	Early stage	≤3 nodules ≤3 cm	Curative Transplant RFA
B	Intermediate stage	Multinodular	Palliative or downstaging to transplant TACE, TARE, other locoregional therapies
C	Advanced stage	Portal invasion or extrahepatic spread	Palliative TACE, TARE Systemic radiation and medical therapies
D	Terminal stage	Incurable widespread or invasive disease	Palliative Systemic medical therapies

Based on his lab and clinical data, our patient is BCLC stage B

The BCLC classification is comprised of five stages (stages 0 and A–D) based upon tumor size, metastasis, performance status, and liver function (based on Child-Pugh score, which grades cirrhosis severity based on total bilirubin, serum albumin, PT or INR, amount of ascites, and hepatic encephalopathy). Patients meeting the requirement for early-stage HCC (BCLC stages 0 and A) are asymptomatic and are good candidates for curative treatment. Patients with intermediate-stage HCC (BCLC stage B) are symptomatic but have preserved liver function. These patients are good candidates for locoregional and systemic therapies. Patients with advanced disease (BCLC stages C–D) have a poor prognosis and are candidates for systemic or palliative therapy. A large longitudinal study found that the median overall survival time was 3.6 months for all untreated HCC. Further, median survival times for untreated HCC with Barcelona Clinic Liver Cancer stages 0/A, B, C, and D were 13.4, 9.5, 3.4, and 1.6 months, respectively.

Question 5. How should HCC treatment decisions ideally be made?

At most large healthcare institutions, HCC treatment decisions are made at a tumor board. A tumor board is a regularly scheduled multidisciplinary conference where each case is presented, and diagnostic and treatment decisions are made in a group setting. The patient's imaging studies are analyzed by radiologists, and potential treatment options are discussed by hepatologists, pathologists, surgeons, radiologists, interventional radiologists, and radiation and medical oncologists. Ancillary services and additional resources available at tumor boards include social workers, nurse navigators, etc. to help implement treatment plans. Tumor boards enable organized collaboration from experts in different fields in order to provide the best treatment for each patient. Studies suggest that the use of tumor boards has led to higher utilization of guideline-recommended curative therapies.

Question 6. What are the treatment options for this lesion?

Many therapeutic options exist, and HCC therapy should be individualized based on the stage (see Table 11.2). In addition to potentially curative surgical treatment, there has been a proliferation of new locoregional and systemic therapies over recent years. Liver transplantation is theoretically the best treatment option, as it will cure both the HCC and the underlying cirrhosis. It is recommended for patients with decompensated cirrhosis. Due to the limited supply of organs, strict and objective eligibility criteria exist to help ensure that livers are allocated to selected individuals with the greatest likelihood of posttransplantation success.

To qualify for liver transplant, patients must first have tumors that fall within the Milan criteria. The Milan criteria are derived from a landmark 1996 study showing >90% recurrence-free survival at 4 years after liver transplant for HCC when lesions in the diseased liver satisfied the following criteria: (1) either a single tumor ≤5 cm or up to three tumors, each ≤3 cm; (2) no evidence of vascular invasion; and (3) no extrahepatic spread (including regional lymph node involvement).

Priority for transplantation is established with Model for End-Stage Liver Disease (MELD) scoring, which predicts 3-month mortality. MELD scores are based on four factors: (1) creatinine, (2) bilirubin, (3) INR, and (4) sodium. In addition, a number of conditions are eligible for additional MELD "exception" upgrade

Table 11.2 HCC treatment modalities

	Mechanism	Notes
Curative treatments		
Surgical resection	Individual tumors are surgically resected	Most appropriate for solitary liver tumors and unilobar disease Reserved for patients with well-preserved liver function Increasing worldwide usage
Liver transplant	Orthotopic liver transplantation	Milan criteria used to identify transplant candidates When meeting Milan criteria, individuals can qualify for MELD exception upgrade points to prioritize transplantation for HCC
Locoregional treatments		
Radiofrequency ablation/microwave ablation	Energy is generated by radio or microwaves which causes tumor necrosis	RFA is considered curative in certain instances Generally preferred for smaller lesions (<3 cm) Limited by tumor proximity to other organs (e.g., bowel)
Transarterial chemoembolization (TACE)	Chemotherapeutic agents are infused into hepatic tissue through percutaneous catheterization of the hepatic artery	Indicated for unresectable lesions Used for tumor downstaging Post-embolization syndrome (fever, right upper quadrant pain, nausea, ileus, elevated liver enzymes) can occur

Table 11.2 (continued)

	Mechanism	Notes
Transarterial radioembolization (TARE)	Radioactive material (resin or glass beads coated with yttrium-90) is infused into the hepatic arteries	Indicated for unresectable lesions Used for tumor downstaging Can be used with portal vein thrombosis More favorable side-effect profile than TACE
Irreversible electroporation (IRE)	Electrical pulses are used to create pores in the cellular membrane of tumor cells	Close proximity of tumor to other organs is not a barrier to use May cause arrhythmias and disruption of cardiac pacemakers
Percutaneous ethanol injection (PEI) and cryoablation	PEI: ethanol is directly injected into tumors Cryoablation: liquid nitrogen or argon gas are used to freeze tumor cells	No longer preferred due to superiority of other locoregional therapies
Radiation therapy	Electromagnetic radiation is used to destroy tumor cells	Appropriate for unresectable lesions
Systemic chemotherapies		
Sorafenib Regorafenib	Oral multikinase inhibitors	Mortality benefit in advanced-stage HCC

points, which are designed to prioritize certain conditions for transplant. Through these exception points, HCC patients who satisfy Milan criteria can be awarded a MELD score of 28 with subsequent 10% increases at 3-month follow-up intervals (to a maximum of 34 points).

Resection takes advantage of the liver's unique ability to regenerate after surgery. Resection is another potentially curative option and one that has traditionally been reserved for patients with solitary liver nodules without vascular invasion and preserved liver function (BCLC stages A–B and Child-Pugh class A).

Locoregional therapies for HCC have evolved rapidly with advances in interventional radiologic techniques. With the exception of radiofrequency ablation (RFA), locoregional therapies are generally not considered curative, but these therapies have proven very successful. The major locoregional treatment modalities are RFA, microwave ablation (MWA), transcatheter arterial chemoembolization (TACE), transarterial radioembolization (TARE), irreversible electroporation (IRE), percutaneous ethanol injection (PEI), and cryoablation. All of these methods require post-procedure imaging and surveillance in order to monitor response and plan additional therapy.

In RFA, alternating current radio waves are applied directly into the tumor by a probe which is inserted either percutaneously or laparoscopically. Thermal energy generated by the radio waves causes tumor necrosis. Solitary lesions smaller than 3 cm are most appropriate for RFA, as it is generally less effective on larger lesions. Multiple studies have demonstrated the efficacy of RFA, and patients within the Milan criteria have 1-year survival rates approaching 97%, 3-year survival rates between 60% and 87%, and 5-year survival rates between 40% and 75%. In MWA, needle electrodes are used to deliver microwave radiation to tumors, typically placed under ultrasound guidance. This modality is also most effective when used on lesions smaller than 3 cm. Response rates of MWA are similar to RFA, and it appears to be a suitable alternative.

In recent years, TACE has become one of the most commonly used therapies for HCC, both for primary therapy and for downstaging (treating tumors with the intent to reduce the size and/or number to meet Milan criteria to allow liver transplant consideration). In this therapy, percutaneous catheterization of the hepatic artery enables chemotherapeutic agents to be infused directly into hepatic tissue. Once infused, an injectable procoagulant is then used to embolize the artery. Tumor necrosis is achieved through direct cytotoxicity from chemotherapy (most often with doxorubicin) and tissue ischemia. There is growing evidence that delivery of cytotoxic agents in the form of drug-eluting beads (DEB-TACE) may be equally efficacious and cause fewer side effects.

TACE is typically considered in well-compensated patients with multifocal HCC or with tumors that are not amenable to resection or ablative therapy. Portal vein thrombosis is a contraindication to TACE due to increased risk of liver failure post-TACE. TACE is usually safe and well tolerated, but significant complications are possible, including liver failure, liver abscess, bile duct injury, and post-embolization syndrome. Post-embolization syndrome is the development of hyperbilirubinemia, elevated transaminases, nausea, right upper quadrant pain, and ileus days to weeks after the procedure.

TARE is a newer treatment modality for HCC which involves infusion of radioactive material into the hepatic arteries that feed tumors. Resin or glass beads coated with yttrium-90 (Y90) are typically used. Studies have shown TARE to be non-inferior to TACE. Unlike TACE, TARE can be used in patients with portal vein thrombosis. TARE also has a more favorable side-effect profile than TACE, leading to less abdominal pain and fewer hospital admissions.

IRE uses electrical pulses to create pores in the cellular membrane of tumor cells, leading to apoptosis and death. It can precisely target tumor cells and causes minimal damage to surrounding tissue. It is thus a good option for tumors in close proximity to vascular structures and other organs. Studies suggest excellent tumor response to IRE, with a 2014 systemic review showing success rates ranging from 67% to 100%.

PEI and cryoablation are now rarely used due to the success of the above locoregional therapies. In addition, the exact role of entities such as external beam radiation therapy (EBRT) and proton beam radiation therapy is being studied.

Systemic chemotherapy is reserved for patients with advanced HCC (BCLC stage C or D). Traditional agents such as doxorubicin, gemcitabine, and oxaliplatin were associated with poor response rates.

Sorafenib, an oral multikinase inhibitor first approved for use in 2007, was the first oral agent to show a survival benefit in HCC. Significant adverse reactions include diarrhea, weight loss, hand-foot-skin eruptions, and hypophosphatemia. Regorafenib is a more powerful oral multikinase inhibitor that was approved in 2017 for patients with advanced-stage HCC who failed treatment with sorafenib. It has a similar side-effect profile to sorafenib. Both medications are recommended for advanced-stage HCC per the AASLD and BCLC treatment guidelines.

Finally, immunotherapy has shown promise in the treatment of HCC. Drugs in this class include nivolumab (anti-PD-1), pembrolizumab (anti-PD-1), tremelimumab (ant-CTLA-4), and ipilimumab (ant-CTLA-4). Clinical trials are currently underway.

Patient Treatment Course

Our patient was discussed at the multidisciplinary tumor board. Based on the specific characteristics of our patient's tumor, DEB-TACE was offered with the goal of downstaging his tumor to meet Milan criteria and allow him to be eligible for liver transplant with MELD exception upgrade points. He had an excellent response to the treatment. After DEB-TACE, his AFP decreased to 8 ng/mL, and imaging studies indicated a significant decrease in tumor size to 2.3 cm. He was eventually awarded the MELD exception upgrade points and underwent a successful liver transplant. He has an excellent short-term prognosis and a moderate long-term prognosis. For patients meeting Milan criteria, 5-year survival is >70% with a recurrence rate of 10–15%. At the time of publication, he continues to do well, with no signs of HCC recurrence.

Conclusions

Hepatocellular carcinoma (HCC) is the most common primary cancer of the liver and generally occurs in patients with underlying cirrhosis. International guidelines generally recommend screening such patients with ultrasound (and AFP) every 6 months. Suspicious lesions should be better characterized with more advanced imaging (such as multiphasic MRI or CT) which can often allow HCC diagnosis without the need for liver biopsy. Once the diagnosis and stage are established, a multidisciplinary approach should be utilized to determine the best individual treatment plan for the patient. Many excellent treatment modalities exist for HCC.

Further Reading

1. Bruix J, Sherman M. Management of hepatocellular carcinoma: an update. Hepatology. 2011;53(3):1020–2.
2. Forner A, Llovet JM, Bruix J. Hepatocellular carcinoma. Lancet. 2012;379:1245–55.
3. Gosalia AJ, Martin P, Jones PD. Advances and future directions in the treatment of hepatocellular carcinoma. Gastroenterol & Hepatol. 2017;13(7):398.
4. Heimbach JK, Kulik LM, Finn RS, Sirlin CB, Abecassis MM, Roberts LR, et al. AASLD guidelines for the treatment of hepatocellular carcinoma. Hepatology. 2018;67(1):358–80.
5. Khalaf N, Ying J, Mittal S, Temple S, Kanwal F, Davila J, El-Serag HB. Natural history of untreated hepatocellular carcinoma in a US

cohort and the role of cancer surveillance. Clin Gastroenterol and Hepatol. 2017;15(2):273–81. e1
6. Mazzaferro V, Regalia E, Doci R, Andreola S, Pulvirenti A, Bozzetti F, et al. Liver transplantation for the treatment of small hepatocellular carcinomas in patients with cirrhosis. N Engl J Med. 1996;334(11):693–700.
7. Mitchell DG, Bruix J, Sherman M, Sirlin CB. LI-RADS (liver imaging reporting and data system): summary, discussion, and consensus of the LI-RADS management working group and future directions. Hepatology. 2015;61(3):1056–65.

Chapter 12
Abnormal Liver Tests

Paul Y. Kwo and Katherine Wong

Introduction

The burden of chronic liver disease continues to increase in the United States. While there have been major achievements in the treatment of certain chronic liver diseases including chronic viral hepatitis, practicing clinicians routinely encounter patients with elevated liver tests. It is important for clinicians to be able to recognize liver tests that are outside the normal range and proceed with a focused evaluation that is tailored to the clinical presentation.

Clinical Case Scenario

A 65-year-old female presents to her primary care provider for a new visit and physical examination. She has a history of diabetes, hyperlipidemia, and osteoarthritis of the back. Her prior surgeries include cesarean section and cholecystectomy. Her medications are metformin, pravastatin, and occasional ibuprofen. She also takes several supplements, including turmeric. Family

P. Y. Kwo (✉) · K. Wong
Stanford University School of Medicine, Palo Alto, CA, USA
e-mail: pkwo@stanford.edu

© Springer Nature Switzerland AG 2019
S. M. Cohen, P. Davitkov (eds.), *Liver Disease*,
https://doi.org/10.1007/978-3-319-98506-0_12

history reveals no known liver disease. There is no tobacco use, and she drinks 1–2 beers per day. There is a remote history of intravenous drug use when she was in her 20s. She denies tattoos. She is married with two adult children. Her BP is 130/80, pulse 70, weight 90 kg, and BMI 34. Her physical examination demonstrates central obesity. Routine laboratory testing reveals glucose 154 mg/dL, alanine aminotransferase (ALT) 85 U/L (with an upper limit of normal <60 U/L), aspartate aminotransferase (AST) 60 U/L (ULN of 45 U/L), alkaline phosphatase 130 U/L (ULN 125 U/L), gamma-glutamyl transferase (GGT) 40 U/L (normal 9–48 U/L), total bilirubin 0.7 mg/dL (ULN of 1.0 mg/dL), albumin 4.0 g/dL (normal 3.5–5.5 g/dL), cholesterol 190 mg/dL, triglycerides 140 mg/dL, WBC 5.0, hemoglobin 14 g/dL, platelets 240,000, and INR 1.0.

Questions

1. How would you characterize her pattern of liver test abnormalities and degree of liver test abnormalities?
2. What confirmatory tests would you like to order?
3. What additional testing should you obtain at this time?
4. What initial recommendations can you make to this patient?

Discussion

Question 1. How would you characterize her pattern of liver test abnormalities and degree of liver test abnormalities?

This patient presents with mildly elevated liver chemistries in a hepatocellular pattern of injury. Hepatocellular injury is defined as a disproportionate elevation of AST and ALT levels as compared with the alkaline phosphatase level. AST and ALT are markers of hepatocellular injury, not liver function. Markers of liver function include albumin, bilirubin, and prothrombin time, and these can be affected by extrahepatic factors. A cholestatic pattern of injury would demonstrate an elevated alkaline phosphatase level that is disproportionately elevated compared to the AST and ALT levels. Our patient has a mildly elevated ALT level that is above the upper limit of normal and thus has a hepatocellular pattern of injury.

Multiple studies across multiple populations have proposed an upper limit of normal for the ALT level either by excluding those with viral hepatitis and elevated BMI, triglycerides, glucose, and cholesterol or by assessing the risk of liver-related mortality with the proposed ULN for ALT ranging from 19 to 25 U/L for females and 29–33 U/L for males. Thus, while our patient's ALT is less than twofold above the ULN for the local lab, it is more than threefold increase above what is considered a true healthy ALT level (19–25 U/L). While these elevations in AST and ALT are mild, they should still be assessed. The 2017 American College of Gastroenterology (ACG) guidelines defined an upper limit of normal for ALT levels and based the evaluation of abnormal ALT levels on the degree of evaluation of ALT. This patient would be in the "mild" elevation category (defined as 2–5X the ULN of ALT). In this chapter, we will focus on our patient with mild ALT and alkaline phosphatase elevations. See Figs. 12.1 and 12.2. The full ACG guidelines outline an approach to patients with various degrees of ALT and AST elevations.

Question 2. What confirmatory tests would you like to order?

Prior to initiating an evaluation of abnormal liver chemistries, one should repeat the liver tests or perform a confirmatory test. In our patient, the ALT was elevated as was the AST level.

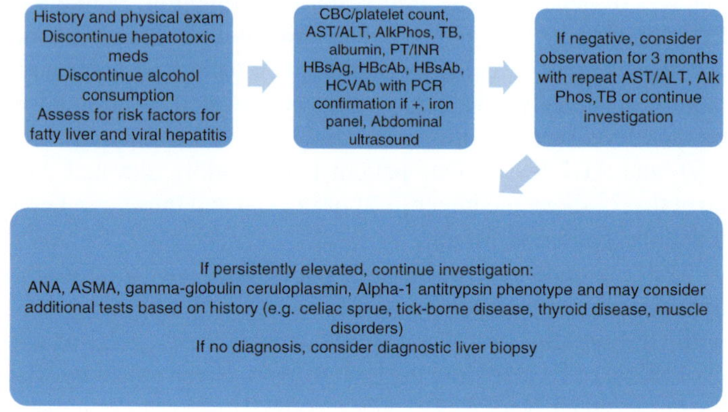

Fig. 12.1 Approach to the patient with a mildly elevated ALT level

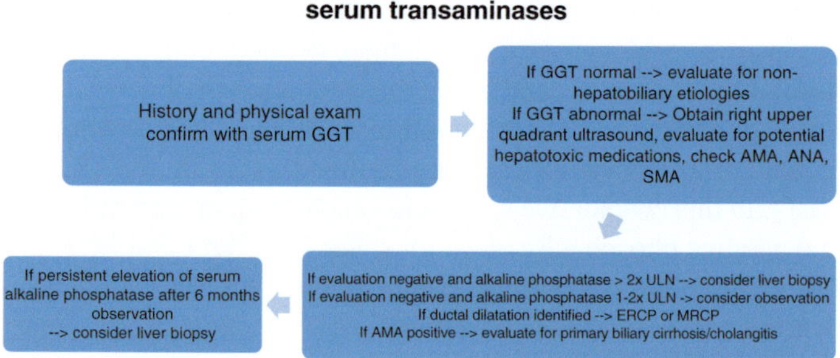

Fig. 12.2 Approach to the patient with an elevated alkaline phosphatase level

This points to a true hepatocellular pattern of elevation. In this patient, prior to proceeding with an evaluation, one could also repeat a liver panel to confirm elevation of ALT and AST. A confirmatory test for elevated alkaline phosphatase is the concomitant elevation of GGT. Alternatively, one could fractionate the alkaline phosphatase level. In a patient with an elevated bilirubin, fractionation of the bilirubin would be the first test ordered. Gilbert's syndrome, a condition affecting 3–7% of the US population, is the most common cause of elevated unconjugated hyperbilirubinemia.

In our patient, the GGT level was normal which suggests that the alkaline phosphatase level elevation is non-hepatic in origin. Given her history of osteoarthritis, the mild elevation in alkaline phosphatase is likely from a bone source. Her serum bilirubin level was normal.

Question 3. What additional testing should you obtain at this time?

The 2017 ACG guideline suggests that the approach to elevated liver tests should be guided by the degree of elevation. Borderline and mild elevations require assessment by the care provider, but an extensive evaluation need not be undertaken initially. In any patient with signs of acute liver failure (prolonged INR with elevated liver tests and hepatic encephalopathy without a prior history of liver disease), immediate referral to a transplant center should be considered.

Our patient has risk factors for multiple chronic liver diseases. Given her history of diabetes and elevated BMI and hyperlipidemia, she is at risk for nonalcoholic fatty liver disease (NAFLD), a condition that affects one third of the US population and approximately one quarter of the world's population. In fact, it is the most common cause of elevated liver tests worldwide. To diagnose NAFLD, one looks for risk factors associated with the metabolic syndrome (which our patient has), and in addition, an ultrasound of the liver should be obtained as part of the evaluation of her elevated ALT level to look for a heterogeneous liver echotexture. Moreover, an ultrasound is relatively inexpensive and can also suggest other features of more advanced liver disease such as splenomegaly (from chronic portal hypertension) or a nodular liver. If NAFLD is suspected, an assessment to determine whether or not the patient has simple steatosis or nonalcoholic steatohepatitis (NASH), which can progress to more advanced fibrosis and cirrhosis, is warranted. The use of transient elastography, serum markers of fibrosis (both commercially available and derived from commonly ordered liver tests such as FIB-4), as well as predictive models such as the NAFLD fibrosis score (http://www.nafldscore.com/) can all be used to noninvasively risk-stratify patients.

Our patient also has risk factors for viral hepatitis with her history of remote IV drug use. The CDC has recommended a one-time hepatitis C virus (HCV) screening test (anti-HCV) for all individuals born between 1945 and 1965. Figure 12.3 outlines the current screening recommendations for HCV. In addition, she should be screened for hepatitis B with a hepatitis B surface antigen test. Finally, hereditary hemochromatosis is a disorder of

One-time HCV testing is recommended for persons born between 1945 and 1965*, without prior ascertainment of risk. Rating: Class I, Level B	Birth cohort screening
• Other persons should be screened for risk factors for HCV infection, and 1-time testing should be performed for all persons with behaviors, exposures, and conditions associated with an increased risk of HCV infection.	Risk-based screening

Risk Behaviors	Exposures	Other

• Injection-drug use (current or ever, including those who injected once)
 	
• Intranasal illicit drug use
	• Long-term hemodialysis (ever)
	• Getting a tattoo in an unregulated setting
	• Health care, emergency medical, and public safety workers after needlesticks, sharps, or mucosal exposures to HCV-infected blood
	• Children born to HCV-infected women
	• Prior recipients of transfusions or organ transplants, including persons who:
	  o Were notified that they received blood from a donor who later tested positive for HCV infection
	  o Received a transfusion of blood or blood components, or underwent an organ transplant before July 1992
	  o Received clotting factor concentrates produced before 1987
	• Persons who were ever incarcerated
		• HIV infection
		• Unexplained chronic liver disease and chronic hepatitis including elevated alanine aminotransferase levels
		
		• Solid organ donors (deceased and living)

Rating: ClassI, Level B

*Regardless of country of birth
AASLD/IDSA Recommendations for Testing, Managing, and Treating Hepatitis C.2015.http://www.hcvguidelines.org/full-report-view. Accessed March 2,2015.

Fig. 12.3 Populations to be tested for hepatitis C

iron absorption and is one of the most common autosomal recessive diseases in Caucasians. There are two classic mutations that occur at the HFE locus for hemochromatosis. The major mutation is C282Y where tyrosine replaces cystine with the minor mutation being H63D where aspartate replaces histidine. If her serum ferritin is elevated and/or transferrin saturation is above 45%, HFE gene analysis should be ordered. It should be noted that elevated ferritin is common in other diseases such as NAFLD, alcoholic liver disease, and viral hepatitis.

Complete serologic evaluation for all causes of elevated liver tests (as outlined in Fig. 12.1) and liver biopsy are usually not initially indicated in the evaluation of minimally or mildly elevated liver enzymes unless laboratory and imaging tests are unrevealing, the abnormalities persist, or there is concern for more advanced disease. If findings of advanced liver disease are revealed, referral to a hepatologist or gastroenterologist is warranted.

Question 4: What initial recommendations can you make to this patient?

In addition to the blood tests that need to be ordered, this patient should be counseled on three specific areas. First, she should be counseled to stop all alcohol use. While her liver chemistry profile is not typical for heavy alcohol use (where one would expect AST > ALT, as well as elevated GGT), she should still stop all alcohol consumption for a period of time until the final etiology of her elevated liver tests is determined. Second, in addition to stopping alcohol, she should stop her supplements such as the turmeric and any potentially hepatotoxic medicines. Complementary or alternative medicines (supplements) may be associated with drug-induced liver injury (DILI), and the clinician should query carefully about the use of any supplements. The three medications she takes are unlikely to be etiologic in her ALT elevation, although statins can elevate ALT and AST levels and are very rarely associated with a cholestatic jaundice. If no other causes for her elevated liver tests are found, temporarily holding the potentially hepatotoxic medicines may be considered though in this case the statin is unlikely to be contributing to her elevated liver tests. Third, lifestyle modifications must be addressed with this patient given her risk factors for NAFLD. Her BMI is 34, she has diabetes, and she has hyperlipidemia. A multidisciplinary effort to lose weight should be undertaken with this patient regardless of the cause of her elevated liver tests.

Additional Clinical Information and Test Results and Interpretation

This patient returns to see you 4 weeks after obtaining additional bloodwork. Her viral hepatitis serologies are negative and her iron panel is normal. She has stopped her turmeric and has ceased all alcohol use. In addition, she has lost three pounds. An ultrasound reveals a heterogeneous liver with a sharp edge and no splenomegaly. Her repeat liver panel shows an AST of 40 U/L and an ALT of 74 U/L. You make a presumptive diagnosis of NAFLD. A NAFLD fibrosis score is calculated and reveals −2.5 which suggests that her risk of advanced fibrosis is low. In addition, a transient elastography test shows no significant fibrosis. You explain to the patient that her pattern of liver enzyme elevation (ALT > AST) indicates NAFLD, but her numbers are now improving with lifestyle modifications. Additionally, her low fibrosis score, normal platelet count, and normal transient elastography indicate that she does not have advanced liver disease. You encourage her to continue with lifestyle modifications. You agree to see her back in 3 months. In the future, should her liver tests fail to normalize, additional testing and even liver biopsy could be considered, as outlined in Fig. 12.1.

Conclusions

Elevated liver enzymes are a common problem encountered in everyday practice. Clinicians need to be aware of a systematic and logical approach to such patients. The clinician should focus on the most likely etiology and tailor their initial workup to such diagnoses. The use of medications (both prescription and over-the-counter) as well as herbal supplements should be considered in the differential diagnosis. Practice guidelines exist to help the clinician in evaluating patients with elevated liver tests.

Further Reading

1. Kwo PY, Cohen SM, Lim JK. ACG clinical guideline: evaluation of abnormal liver chemistries. Am J Gastroenterol. 2017;112:18–35.
2. Udompap P, Kim D, Kim WR. Current and future burden of chronic non-malignant liver disease. Clin Gastroenterol Hepatol. 2015;13:2031–41.
3. Chalasani N, et al. The diagnosis and management of nonalcoholic fatty liver disease: practice guidance from the American Association for the Study of Liver Diseases. Hepatology. 2018;67:328–57.
4. CDC guidelines on HCV screening. https://www.cdc.gov/hepatitis/hcv/guidelinesc.htm. Accessed 30 May 2018
5. AASLD/IDSA Recommendations for Testing, Managing, and Treating Hepatitis C. 2015. http://www.hcvguidelines.org/full-report-view. Accessed 2 Mar 2015.
6. Dutta A, Saha C, Johnson CS, et al. Variability in the upper limit of normal for serum alanine aminotransferase levels: a statewide study. Hepatology. 2009;50:1957–62.
7. Ruhl CE, Everhart JE. Elevated serum alanine aminotransferase and gamma-glutamyltransferase and mortality in the United States population. Gastroenterology. 2009;136:477–85.

Chapter 13
General Care of the Cirrhotic Patient

Paul A. Schmeltzer and Mark W. Russo

Introduction

Cirrhosis is the end stage of a wide variety of chronic liver diseases. It is a histologic term defined by the presence of fibrous septa throughout the liver that divide the hepatic parenchyma into nodules. Clinically, patients can be classified as having compensated or decompensated disease. Compensated cirrhosis implies that the liver can perform vital functions normally. Hepatic decompensation, which is characterized by ascites, variceal bleeding, or hepatic encephalopathy, markedly affects life expectancy. Cirrhosis is a major public health problem; it was the 8th leading cause of death in the USA in 2010. This chapter will describe a case of compensated cirrhosis. We will address the aspects of general cirrhosis care that are important for primary care physicians.

P. A. Schmeltzer
Department of Hepatology, Carolinas Medical Center,
Charlotte, NC, USA

M. W. Russo (✉)
Carolinas Medical Center, Charlotte, NC, USA
e-mail: mark.russo@carolinashealthcare.org

© Springer Nature Switzerland AG 2019
S. M. Cohen, P. Davitkov (eds.), *Liver Disease*,
https://doi.org/10.1007/978-3-319-98506-0_13

Clinical Case Scenario

A 55-year-old male with class 1 obesity, insulin-dependent diabetes mellitus, hypertension, and dyslipidemia returns to his primary care physician after undergoing a laparoscopic cholecystectomy for symptomatic cholelithiasis. His surgeon noted a nodular liver during the operation, consistent with cirrhosis. His physical exam is only notable for obesity. There are no stigmata of chronic liver disease. His medications include metoprolol, metformin, and atorvastatin. He reports rare alcohol use. Past labs show intermittent, mild aminotransferase elevations, mild thrombocytopenia (platelets 125,000), INR 1.0, serum sodium 140 mmol/L, creatinine 0.6 mg/dL, and a bilirubin of 1.0 mg/dL. A preoperative right upper quadrant ultrasound showed hepatic steatosis and cholelithiasis without biliary duct dilation.

Questions

1. What is the etiology of this patient's cirrhosis?
2. How should a cirrhotic be screened for hepatocellular carcinoma?
3. How should a cirrhotic patient be screened for gastroesophageal varices?
4. What immunizations should a cirrhotic patient receive?
5. Can a cirrhotic patient take atorvastatin?
6. What nutritional recommendations should be provided to a patient with NAFLD cirrhosis?
7. What is the prognosis of a cirrhotic patient and when should a referral for liver transplant be made?

Discussion

Question 1. What is the etiology of this patient's cirrhosis?

Cirrhosis can develop from many different causes including chronic viral hepatitis, autoimmune disorders, inherited disorders, alcohol use, and metabolic disease such as nonalcoholic fatty liver disease (NAFLD) or nonalcoholic steatohepatitis (NASH). It is important to determine the etiology of cirrhosis as certain treatments may prevent further liver injury. Oftentimes a diagnosis can be made based on clinical history and serologies alone. Histopathologic findings in a cirrhotic are frequently non-specific. A liver biopsy may be helpful if there is a concern for active autoimmune hepatitis, Wilson disease, or alcoholic liver disease when the clinical history is uncertain. However, a liver biopsy is frequently not needed to determine the etiology of cirrhosis, which in most cases can be determined from history, physical exam, and blood work. A list of lab tests and corresponding clinical clues is provided below (see Table 13.1).

The following serologies were obtained on our patient:

Hepatitis A total antibody: Negative
Hepatitis B surface antigen: Negative
Hepatitis B surface antibody: Positive
Hepatitis C antibody: Negative
Antinuclear antibody: Negative
Antimitochondrial antibody: Negative
Smooth muscle antibody: Negative
Serum immunoglobulins: Negative
Ferritin: 300 micrograms per liter
Transferrin saturation: 35%
Alpha-1 antitrypsin phenotype: MM

Table 13.1 Chronic liver disease evaluation

Disease	Screening test(s)	Clinical clue(s)
Hepatitis C	Hepatitis C (HCV) antibody	Viral hepatitis risk factors, baby boomers (born from 1945 to 1965)
Hepatitis B	Hepatitis B surface antigen (HBsAg)	Viral hepatitis risk factors, mother with hepatitis B
Alcoholic liver disease	None	2:1 AST to ALT ratio
NAFLD	None	Metabolic syndrome
Autoimmune hepatitis	Antinuclear antibody (ANA), smooth muscle antibody (SMA), IgG	Young woman with other autoimmune conditions
Primary biliary cholangitis	Antimitochondrial antibody (AMA)	Middle-aged/elderly female with cholestasis
Primary sclerosing cholangitis	MRCP/ERCP	Cholestasis, history of inflammatory bowel disease (IBD)
Hereditary hemochromatosis	Ferritin, transferrin saturation, genetic hemochromatosis test	Elderly male, diabetes, arthritis, family history of iron overload
Alpha-1 antitrypsin deficiency	A1AT level/phenotype	
Wilson disease	Ceruloplasmin, 24-h copper	Young patient, hemolysis, neuropsychiatric disease
Budd Chiari	Doppler ultrasound	Hypercoagulable disorder, ascites

The elevated ferritin with a normal transferrin saturation is not consistent with hereditary hemochromatosis. Ferritin may be elevated in 30–50% of patients with viral hepatitis, alcoholic liver disease, and NAFLD. Given the patient's clinical history and above lab results, his cirrhosis is likely due to NAFLD. A liver biopsy is unlikely to provide additional information since labs do not suggest a coexisting cause of chronic liver disease.

The patient is provided counseling regarding weight loss and exercise. Studies have shown that a 7–10% reduction of body weight can improve steatosis and fibrosis. Going forward, it will also be important for him to have good control of his metabolic comorbidities (diabetes, dyslipidemia, hypertension). There are no effective FDA-approved pharmacologic therapies for NAFLD at this time. However, phase 3 trials are being conducted on agents including obeticholic acid (a farnesoid X receptor agonist) and elafibranor (a PPAR α/δ agonist).

Question 2. How should a cirrhotic patient be screened for hepatocellular carcinoma?

The incidence rate of hepatocellular carcinoma (HCC) in cirrhotics is 2–4% per year. An Asian study of patients with hepatitis B showed a 37% reduction in mortality for those who underwent HCC surveillance. This survival benefit is thought to occur due to detection of earlier stage disease that can lead to curative treatment.

The American Association for the Study of Liver Diseases (AASLD) has established guidelines for HCC surveillance and treatment. Surveillance with ultrasound every 6 months is recommended. The addition of serum alpha-fetoprotein (AFP) every 6 months is considered optional. AFP has a low sensitivity for the detection of early stage HCC, and it is not clear that its use adds to the performance characteristics of ultrasound. This author incorporates AFP into HCC surveillance in part because the prevalence of NASH is increasing in the US population and ultrasound can be suboptimal in obese patients.

It is important to mention that certain non-cirrhotic hepatitis B (HBV)-infected patients should undergo HCC screening as well. These include HBV-infected Asian men over 40 years old, Asian women over 50 years old, Africans over 20 years old, and persons with a first-degree family member with a history of HCC.

The patient in the scenario above had an ultrasound prior to his recent cholecystectomy that did not show any liver masses. His AFP was normal at 2 ng/mL. His future surveillance for HCC will include AFP and ultrasound every 6 months.

Question 3. How should a cirrhotic patient be screened for gastroesophageal varices?

Esophageal varices develop in more than one third of patients with cirrhosis within 3 years of diagnosis. Variceal formation is the result of fibrosis in the hepatic sinusoids that generates portal hypertension. Factors that influence variceal bleeding include the size of the varix, the thickness of the varix wall, and the pressure difference between the varix and the esophageal lumen. Measuring transjugular hepatic venous pressures is a way to quantify the degree of portal hypertension, although this is not performed routinely in the US. Varices develop when there is clinically significant portal hypertension (hepatic venous pressure gradient ≥ 10 mmHg), and bleeding occurs when the gradient is ≥ 12 mmHg.

In lieu of invasive testing such as transjugular pressure measurements, noninvasive assessments of liver fibrosis and portal hypertension can be obtained with transient elastography. Clinically significant portal hypertension is suggested by transient elastography scores of >20–25 kPa. The platelet count is another surrogate marker of portal hypertension; large varices are generally not present with a platelet count >150,000. In fact, a low platelet count is a common initial finding of patients with cirrhosis and portal hypertension that may initially be interpreted as idiopathic thrombocytopenia. A compensated cirrhotic with a combined transient elastography measurement of <20 kPa and platelet count >150,000 has a < 5% chance of having large varices and can likely forego screening upper endoscopy.

The patient in the above scenario is compensated but has a platelet count that is <150,000. An EGD is performed and shows large esophageal varices. By definition, he has clinically significant portal hypertension, and primary prophylaxis for variceal hemorrhage is indicated. Options for prophylaxis include nonselective beta-blockers (NSBBs) and variceal band ligation. Since he is already tolerating metoprolol for hypertension, it would be appropriate to switch him to a NSBB such as propranolol, nadolol, or carvedilol. His metoprolol is stopped, and he is started on nadolol 40 mg daily with a goal resting heart rate of 55–60/min. If he had difficulty to control ascites, then the nonselective beta-blocker may need to be discontinued.

Question 4. What immunizations should a cirrhotic patient receive?

Infection in cirrhotic patients is common and significantly affects mortality. While most of these infections are bacterial, superimposed viral infections are important also, and immunizations can help prevent them. Immunizations should be addressed early on during the course of chronic liver disease as they lose their effectiveness as cirrhosis progresses. Inactivated or killed-type vaccinations should be chosen over live attenuated ones. Therefore, the MMR, polio, smallpox, varicella, and live influenza vaccine should not be given to patients with advanced fibrosis/cirrhosis.

The influenza vaccine is safe and effective in compensated cirrhosis, decompensated cirrhosis, and post liver transplant. However, the rate of seroprotection is lower than in healthy controls. The symptoms of influenza may be atypical in cirrhotic patients so immunization is a good preventive measure. The live virus influenza vaccination should not be given to cirrhotics or liver transplant recipients. Standard guidelines for the Pneumovax23 vaccination in immunocompromised hosts apply to patients with chronic liver diseases. Of note, PCV13 is recommended for adults >19 years of age with immunocompromising conditions, but the United States Advisory Committee on Immunization Practices did not consider cirrhosis to fall into this category. Hepatitis A superinfection in patients with chronic liver disease carries a 23-fold risk of death. Seroconversion is achieved in 98% of compensated cirrhotics and 66% of decompensated cirrhotics after the booster dose is given. In healthy individuals, the standard dose hepatitis B vaccine results in a > 90% seroprotective response. This rate decreases to 16–20% in cirrhotics. Administering a double dose of the vaccine at standard intervals can increase the response rate to 68%.

The patient in the above case is immune to hepatitis B. He should be vaccinated against hepatitis A, influenza, and pneumococcus.

Question 5. Can a cirrhotic patient take atorvastatin?

Prior to his cirrhosis diagnosis, this patient was taking atorvastatin for dyslipidemia. Is it safe to continue this medication?

There is a strong association between NAFLD and cardiovascular disease. Cardiovascular disease is the primary cause of death in this population. Studies including the GREek Atorvastatin and Coronary-heart-disease Evaluation (GREACE) study have shown that statins improve aminotransferases and cardiovascular outcomes in patients with elevated liver enzymes presumably due to NAFLD.

The risk of significant hepatotoxicity from statins is very low. One to three percent of patients develop mild, asymptomatic aminotransferase elevations that often resolve with continued statin use. Less than 1% of patients develop aminotransferases above

3 times the upper limit of normal. The risk of statin-induced liver failure is estimated to be 0.2–1 cases per million persons taking statins. The Drug-Induced Liver Injury Network reported only 22 cases of drug-induced liver injury from statins over an 8-year period. Therefore, the risk/benefit ratio favors statin use in a compensated cirrhotic. The AASLD guidelines on NAFLD recommend avoiding statins in decompensated cirrhotics, although often dyslipidemia improves with decompensated disease.

Question 6. What nutritional recommendations should be provided to a patient with NAFLD cirrhosis?

As mentioned earlier, lifestyle modification including weight loss is recommended for patients with NAFLD. A reduction in caloric intake by 500–1000 kcal/day along with increased physical activity is recommended. There is not enough data at this time to recommend one particular macronutrient diet (i.e., Mediterranean diet) over another. Bariatric surgery has been shown to improve some histologic features of NAFLD including steatosis, ballooning, and even fibrosis in 33% of patients based on retrospective and prospective cohort studies. The safety and efficacy of bariatric surgery in NASH cirrhotics has not been well studied. Bariatric surgery would not be recommended for the patient in this clinical vignette because of the presence of clinically significant portal hypertension.

Dietary recommendations may change as a patient's cirrhosis progresses. Malnutrition develops in 20–60% of cirrhotics and the loss of skeletal mass (sarcopenia) is of particular concern. Sarcopenia has been associated with a higher risk of infection and worse posttransplant outcomes. NAFLD patients can have sarcopenia in the setting of obesity. In the past, protein restriction was recommended in cirrhotics to help treat hepatic encephalopathy.

More recent studies have found that protein restriction does not help with hepatic encephalopathy and current guidelines recommend a daily protein intake of 1.2–1.5 g/kg/d. When cirrhotic patients develop ascites, a 2000 mg daily sodium limit is advised. As cirrhosis advances and hyponatremia develops, fluid restriction may be instituted when the serum sodium is less than 120–125 mmol/L.

Question 7. What is the prognosis of a cirrhotic patient, and when should a referral for liver transplant be made?

As mentioned earlier, the two pertinent clinical stages of cirrhosis are (1) compensated and (2) decompensated. The median survival time with compensated cirrhosis is >12 years, whereas it is <2 years with decompensated cirrhosis. The presence of clinically significant portal hypertension is notable as this increases the 1-year mortality in a compensated cirrhotic from <1% to 3–4%.

In addition to monitoring for hepatic decompensation, scoring systems such as the Child-Pugh score and Model for End-Stage Liver Disease (MELD) score are important for determining mortality. The Child-Pugh score was developed to assess mortality risk in patients with cirrhosis undergoing vascular surgery and portosystemic shunt surgery for variceal bleeding. The scoring is based on bilirubin, INR, albumin, severity of ascites, and severity of hepatic encephalopathy. The Child-Pugh score has largely been supplanted by the MELD and sodium-MELD scores which look at INR, creatinine, bilirubin, and sodium. MELD and sodium-MELD accurately predict 3-month mortality in patients awaiting liver transplantation. While there are regional differences in MELD score and time to transplant, it is reasonable to refer a patient to a liver transplant center when they develop hepatic decompensation and/or their MELD score is 15 or higher.

In addition to severity of liver disease, other factors including age, medical comorbidities, and psychosocial factors determine a patient's transplant candidacy and are an important part of a multidisciplinary liver transplant evaluation (Fig. 13.1).

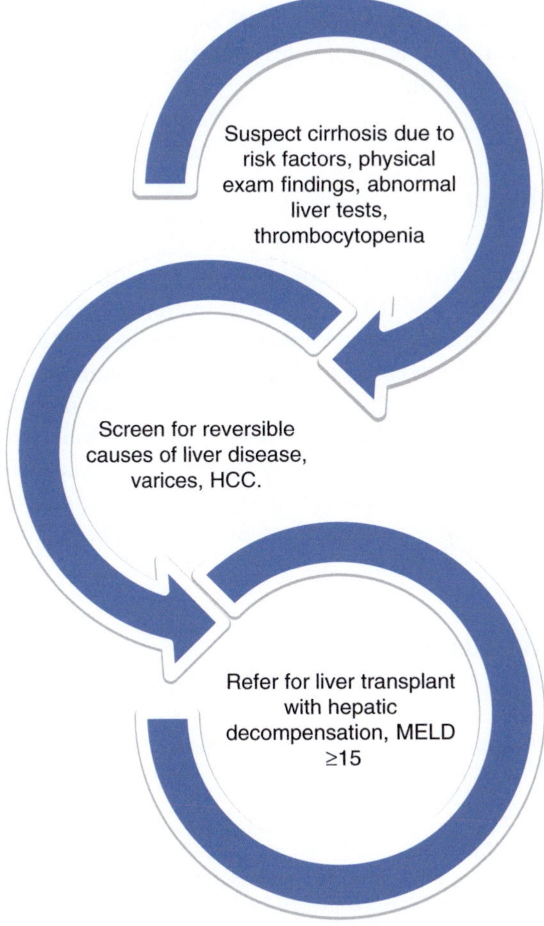

Fig. 13.1 Management of the cirrhotic patient

The patient in the above scenario is early for consideration of transplant based on symptoms and MELD score. He will likely decompensate during his lifetime and likely require a liver transplant evaluation eventually. Because there is a strong association between NASH and cardiovascular disease, cardiovascular testing would be an important part of his transplant evaluation. Posttransplant outcomes for NASH are good with 1- and 3-year patient and graft survival rates comparable to transplant outcomes for other indications.

Conclusions

In summary, cirrhosis is a common disease with a variety of etiologies, some of which have specific treatments that can prevent or halt the progression to decompensated disease. Patients with cirrhosis need screening for hepatocellular carcinoma and may need variceal screening at certain intervals. Care must be taken to avoid certain medications, toxins, or infections that could exacerbate liver disease. In the event of decompensation or worsening liver synthetic function or liver cancer development, a referral to a liver transplant center may be indicated.

Further Reading

1. Chalasani N, Younossi Z, Lavine JE, et al. The diagnosis and management of nonalcoholic fatty liver disease: practice guidance from the American Association for the study of liver diseases. Hepatology. 2018;67(1):328–57.
2. Garcia-Tsao G, Abraldes JG, Berzigotti A, et al. Portal hypertensive bleeding in cirrhosis: risk stratification, diagnosis, and management: 2016 practice guidelines by the American Association for the study of liver diseases. Hepatology. 2017;65(1):310–33.

3. Ge PS, Runyon BA. Treatment of patients with cirrhosis. NEJM. 2016;375(8):767–77.
4. Heimbach JK, Kulik LM, Finn RS, et al. AASLD guidelines for the treatment of hepatocellular carcinoma. Hepatology. 2018;67(1):358–80.
5. Leise MD, Talwalkar JA. Immunizations in chronic liver disease: what should be done and what is the evidence. Curr Gastroenterol Rep. 2013;15:300.

Chapter 14
Hepatic Encephalopathy

Eric Kallwitz and Zurabi Lominadze

Introduction

Hepatic encephalopathy (HE) describes the alteration in brain function that occurs in the setting of advanced liver dysfunction or shunting of blood from the portal to systemic circulation. As such, it represents one of the complications of cirrhosis and portal hypertension. HE can manifest as either subclinical (minimal HE) or overt clinical disease, ranging from mild cognitive impairment to coma. The lifetime risk of overt HE in a cirrhotic patient approaches 30–40%. The presence of HE often has a significant impact on the quality of life of patients and their caregivers, frequently resulting in repeated hospitalizations. Symptoms of liver dysfunction, such as HE, are important as these events signify hepatic decompensation. The degree of HE is incorporated into the Child-Pugh classification of severity of

E. Kallwitz
Division of Hepatology, Department of Medicine, Loyola University Chicago Stritch School of Medicine, Maywood, IL, USA
e-mail: ekallwitz@lumc.edu

Z. Lominadze
Division of Gastroenterology and Nutrition, Department of Medicine, Loyola University Chicago Stritch School of Medicine, Maywood, IL, USA

© Springer Nature Switzerland AG 2019

179

S. M. Cohen, P. Davitkov (eds.), *Liver Disease*,
https://doi.org/10.1007/978-3-319-98506-0_14

liver disease. However, HE is not a part of the Model for End-Stage Liver Disease (MELD) scoring system, which is now the most common and accepted method to assess severity of liver disease. This chapter will focus on the diagnosis and management of HE in the setting of cirrhosis.

Clinical Case Scenario

A 62-year-old female presents to the emergency department. She has a diagnosis of nonalcoholic fatty liver disease and cirrhosis. Her disease has been managed in an outpatient clinic up to this point. Her manifestations of liver disease have included mild fluid overload and ascites which have responded to low doses of furosemide and spironolactone. Her labs reveal total bilirubin of 1.9 mg/dL, international normalized ratio (INR) of 1.4, creatinine of 1.7 mg/dL, and serum sodium of 134 mmol/L. Her MELD-sodium score is 20. She was seen 1 month prior in clinic for chronic disease management with a MELD-Na of 14 and underwent a liver ultrasound which showed no ascites and no evidence of liver cancer. Her husband now brings her to the emergency room and reports that she was a little slow mentally the past few days, often repeating statements. She also has not been eating well recently. Last night she awoke from sleep to use the bathroom, and her husband found her staring at the sink, seemingly unable to turn the faucet on. She only stared with a blank expression when he asked her what was wrong. At the hospital, she is mildly tachycardiac and appears dehydrated. She has no clinical or laboratory findings of infection or bleeding.

Questions

1. How does HE develop?
2. How is HE diagnosed?
3. What are the typical clinical manifestations of HE?
4. How is HE best managed?
5. How should patients with difficult-to-manage HE be approached?

Discussion

Question 1. How does HE develop?

The pathogenesis of HE is complex and incompletely understood. A simplistic way to view the development of HE separates its pathogenesis into factors related to liver dysfunction and factors related to circulatory dysfunction (portal to systemic shunting). Although generally considered reversible, repeated episodes of HE are associated with some degree of chronic and cumulative cognitive deficits, which may persist even after liver transplant.

Liver Dysfunction

Although the changes of HE cannot solely be attributed to the hyperammonemia of liver dysfunction, the impaired metabolism of ammonia is an important contributor to its pathogenesis. Elevated ammonia levels cause increased GABAergic tone, astrocyte dysfunction, and subsequent impaired uptake of glutamate in the brain, resulting in an imbalance between excitatory and inhibitory neurotransmitters. Decreased clearance of other nitrogenous substances from the colon by a dysfunctional liver may also play a role in the development of HE.

Circulatory Dysfunction

In addition to a poorly functioning liver, patients with cirrhosis often have spontaneous portosystemic shunts, allowing substances such as ammonia, inflammatory cytokines, and endotoxin from the gastrointestinal tract to bypass the liver and directly enter the systemic circulation. The significance of such shunting is evident in the fact that HE occurs in about 30% of patients after transjugular intrahepatic portosystemic shunt (TIPS). A growing body of evidence also points to the role of gut microbial dysbiosis in liver dysfunction and HE. Specifically, impaired bile acid synthesis by a poorly functioning liver may lead to deleterious changes in the gut microbiome, while portosystemic shunting allows potentially toxic gut-derived products direct access to the systemic circulation and thus the brain. Advancing liver disease may be associated with an unfavorable shift in the ratio of autochthonous (commensal and potentially beneficial bacteria) to non-autochthonous bacteria, which correlates with increasing MELD score and endotoxin levels.

Question 2. How is HE diagnosed?

HE remains a clinical diagnosis. The diagnosis can be reached by using a stepwise approach, as follows:

1. Does the patient have liver disease or portosystemic shunting? Some features of liver disease or portosystemic shunting should be present to make a diagnosis of HE. History,

physical examination, and imaging can be helpful in this regard. This can include, but is not limited to, the following:

(a) History: known diagnosis of liver disease, family history of liver disease, risk factors for viral hepatitis, risk factors for fatty liver disease, medication use, substance abuse, alcohol abuse

(b) Physical examination: jaundice, spider angiomata, palmar erythema, splenomegaly, ascites, dilated abdominal wall blood vessels, asterixis (described below)

(c) Laboratories: thrombocytopenia indicative of portal hypertension, hyperbilirubinemia, coagulopathy, elevated aminotransferases (although liver enzymes can be normal in cirrhosis)

(d) Imaging: reversal of flow (hepatofugal flow) in the portal vein on ultrasound, contrast imaging (CT or MRI scan) showing collateral vessels or varices

2. Is there another cause of altered mental status?

(a) History: substance use, alcohol use, medication history (including narcotics, sedatives, anticholinergics, and sleep aides), fever, new-onset focal neurologic symptoms

(b) Physical examination: detailed physical examination with detailed neurologic examination

(c) Laboratory testing: complete blood count, complete metabolic panel, urinalysis, cultures when appropriate, toxicology tests

(d) Other tests: imaging of the central nervous system and electroencephalogram when appropriate

3. Does the patient respond as expected to therapy? Improvement of HE symptoms with treatment is expected and often occurs rapidly. If there is a lack of response to therapy, the healthcare provider should consider if the diagnosis of HE is correct. Other causes of altered mental status such as delirium or Wernicke-Korsakoff syndrome can manifest similarly to HE.

Asterixis is often present with hepatic encephalopathy. Asterixis can be assessed by having the patient maintain their hands in a fully extended position. With asterixis, a flap of the fingers in a downward or more flexed position will occur. Asterixis should not be confused with a resting or intention tremor. However, asterixis can be present in other forms of encephalopathy also, so its presence supports the diagnosis of HE only in the appropriate clinical context.

Measuring ammonia levels is sometimes performed when the diagnosis of HE is in question. In this setting, an elevated ammonia level can support the diagnosis, but ammonia levels should not be sent for the intention of making a diagnosis of HE. Additionally, ammonia levels should not be measured serially or used to guide medical therapy in the setting of overt HE. Current guidelines for the management of HE state that ammonia levels do not add diagnostic, prognostic, or staging information. The guidelines do suggest that a normal ammonia level should prompt reevaluation of the diagnosis of HE. Treating a patient based on ammonia levels alone may result in "over-treating" a patient with normal mentation, which can result in volume depletion and electrolyte abnormalities with subsequent worsening of confusion.

Question 3. What are the typical clinical manifestations of HE?

The manifestations of HE can be classified in different manners (Table 14.1). It is important to note that cerebral edema with the risk of cerebral herniation and brain death can occur in the setting of HE associated with acute liver failure (Type A). However, cerebral edema and its associated morbidity/mortality is *not* seen with HE related to chronic liver disease or portosystemic shunting (Types C and B).

Table 14.1 Classifications and common manifestations of hepatic encephalopathy

Classification	Subclassifications	Manifestations
Underlying liver disease	Type A. Acute liver failure	Can be associated with elevated intracranial pressure and cerebral herniation
	Type B. Portosystemic shunting	See additional classifications below
	Type C. Cirrhosis	
HE severity	Minimal	Usually diagnosed through neuropsychiatric testing
	Grade I	Subtle changes, patient or caregiver may notice mild deterioration in cognition or attention
	Grade II	Disorientation and asterixis develops
	Grade III	Gross disorientation and confusion along with somnolence
	Grade IV	Coma, no response to any stimuli
HE time course	Episodic	Infrequent occurrences
	Recurrent	Multiple bouts
	Persistent	Always some alteration, possible periodic worsening
HE precipitants	Non-precipitated	No cause found
	Precipitated	Cause, such as infection or bleeding, found

Modified from Vilstrup et al. *Hepatology*. 2014;60(2):715–35 [12] and Ferenci et al. *Hepatology*. 2002;35:716 [7]

Minimal HE

It is important to be aware of minimal HE. By definition, there are no easily recognizable changes in mentation in this condition. Patients will present alert and oriented and will not have asterixis. However, despite the absence of overt manifestations, minimal HE can still impact patient well-being. Historical clues that physicians should be aware of include patients reporting decreased performance in usual daily tasks or recent motor vehicle accidents. For example, a patient who works as an accountant may report making unusual errors when preparing tax returns. Evaluation for the presence of minimal HE can be done through neuropsychiatric testing or through computer-based programs. Management could include a medication trial. The assessment for a therapeutic effect of medication is sometimes based on patient-reported symptoms but may require more formal repetitive testing.

Overt HE

Overt HE is more easily recognized and includes both neurologic and psychiatric manifestations. In general, patients can be staged using the West Haven criteria of altered mental state in HE and the Glasgow Coma Scale. Grade I HE is characterized by a decrease in attention span and awareness. Alterations or reversals in the sleep-wake cycle can be common and may be the initial manifestation of HE in some patients. Asterixis may be present in Grade I HE, but is not required. Grade II HE is characterized by more notable changes in awareness, and lethargy may be present. Personality changes and abnormal behaviors can also become prominent. At this point, asterixis should be evident. Grade III HE is notable for a somnolent state where it can be difficult to arouse the patient. He or she may not be able to participate in an examination to display asterixis, but the clinician may note muscle rigidity. As HE progresses, the patient may be unable to safely swallow medications. Grade IV is the onset of coma. The Glasgow Coma Scale scores eye opening, motor response, and verbal response.

Clinical Case: Continued

In the emergency room, the patient is diagnosed with HE in the setting of volume depletion. Fluids are given intravenously and lactulose is started. She has four bowel movements over the next 12 h. After a night in observation, her creatinine and sodium have normalized and she is back to her baseline. She is discharged home on lactulose and instructed to follow up with her outpatient physician. She does well for a few months before returning to the emergency department with recurrent symptoms of HE. Her husband reports that she had been doing well on lactulose until the day prior. She was more sleepy than usual during the daytime, was not eating as well, and refused her lactulose on multiple occasions. On this visit, she is diagnosed with a urinary tract infection. Her HE improves after hydration, treatment of the urinary tract infection, and continued lactulose. She is discharged home after a short stay in the hospital, and rifaximin is added to her outpatient medications.

Question 4. How is HE best managed?

Supportive Treatment

If a reversible underlying etiology that triggers HE is found, such as infection, volume depletion, or electrolyte abnormalities, it should be promptly treated. Evaluation for infection should be thorough and include history, examination, and laboratory findings. Spontaneous bacterial peritonitis is a common infection that can result in worsened HE. Therefore, patients with ascites should undergo a diagnostic paracentesis with, at a minimum, cell count and culture. Urinary tract and respiratory tract infections are other potential sources which should be excluded. An evaluation for gastrointestinal bleeding as a trigger for HE should also be considered. Constipation can also result in HE, and it is important to assess with the patient and caregivers how many bowel movements were occurring prior to the development of clinical symptoms. Medication adherence should be assessed, as lactulose has significant side effects that may limit adherence, but the clinician should avoid the temptation to immediately blame "medication non-compliance" as the culprit for recurrent HE episodes.

Euvolemia should be achieved, and any deranged electrolytes, especially hypokalemia, hypomagnesemia, and hypo- or hypernatremia should be corrected. If the patient is comatose and there is concern for inadequate airway protection and the risk of aspiration, the patient should be monitored in an intensive care unit setting and consideration given to intubation.

There should be a low threshold to initiate a nutritional assessment, and small frequent meals plus a bedtime snack should be recommended. There is no role for protein restriction in the treatment of HE. Rather, a goal of 1.2–1.5 g/kg/day of protein intake should be targeted in these patients, and if this cannot be achieved by standard means, oral branched-chain amino acid supplementation can be considered.

As one of the heralding events of decompensated cirrhosis, the onset of HE in a patient should lead to referral to a liver transplant center.

Pharmacologic Treatment

Lactulose remains the mainstay for management of acute overt HE. Doses should be given with a goal of achieving four to five bowel movements daily to treat active HE requiring hospitalization, followed by maintenance dosing to achieve three to four soft bowel movements daily. If the patient is unable to safely swallow medications, a nasogastric tube should be promptly placed to allow safe medication administration. For grades III–IV HE, rectal lactulose via enemas could also be considered. It is important to recognize that after the treatment of an initial episode of HE, long-term maintenance therapy should be instituted. Rifaximin twice daily could be added to lactulose to prevent a recurrent episode of HE. The role of probiotics for HE is not well defined currently, though emerging evidence suggests that they may be of similar efficacy to lactulose for minimal or low-grade HE. Similarly, zinc supplementation is of uncertain benefit.

Both neomycin and metronidazole are accepted alternative treatment options for overt HE. Neomycin was widely used in the past but has been supplanted by lactulose and rifaximin for most cases as it has known risks of ototoxicity and nephrotoxicity. Similarly, a short course of metronidazole may be used in lieu of the previously discussed medications, but its use is also limited due to ototoxicity, nephrotoxicity, and neurotoxicity. In addition, the well-known disulfiram-like reaction that ingestion of alcohol can elicit with metronidazole must be taken into account, especially in patients with alcohol abuse.

In some settings when liver recovery occurs, it may be appropriate to reduce or stop therapy; however, this must be done cautiously and with careful monitoring for recurrence of HE.

Clinical Case: Continued

Unfortunately, despite home use of lactulose and rifaximin, the patient continues to have hospitalizations for HE. Her husband brings her to all scheduled clinic visits and reports adherence with both lactulose and rifaximin. He has taken a leave of absence from his job and is frustrated as he feels that some healthcare staff members are blaming him for the repeated hospitalizations. He is exhausted and reports that he is afraid to leave the house even to go to the store. In addition, he sets an alarm every night for 3 AM to wake her up and give her lactulose. She comes to the appointment in a wheelchair and has lost considerable muscle mass. She has been evaluated and listed for liver transplant, but has not had MELD scores high enough to result in an organ offer. Her husband is wondering what he should do next.

Question 5. How should patients with difficult-to-manage HE be approached?

Refractory HE, whether a single difficult-to-treat episode, or discrete episodes that recur repeatedly with minimal or no obvious precipitating factor, should prompt an evaluation for an alternative cause of altered mental status. If other etiologies for the clinical presentation are excluded, the presence of portosystemic shunts should be considered. In patients with TIPS in this situation, downsizing should be considered, although there is no universally agreed-upon portal pressure to target, and the risks of recurrent varices or ascites must be considered. For patients without TIPS, imaging such as contrast-enhanced CT or MRI may help discover spontaneous portosystemic shunts (Fig. 14.1). Embolization of these shunts by an interventional radiology team may help reduce the frequency and severity of HE. Ultimately, liver transplantation is the only definitive treatment for refractory HE.

For all cases of HE, patient and provider education on early recognition of symptoms, aggressive outpatient treatment, and knowing when to seek help are of paramount importance.

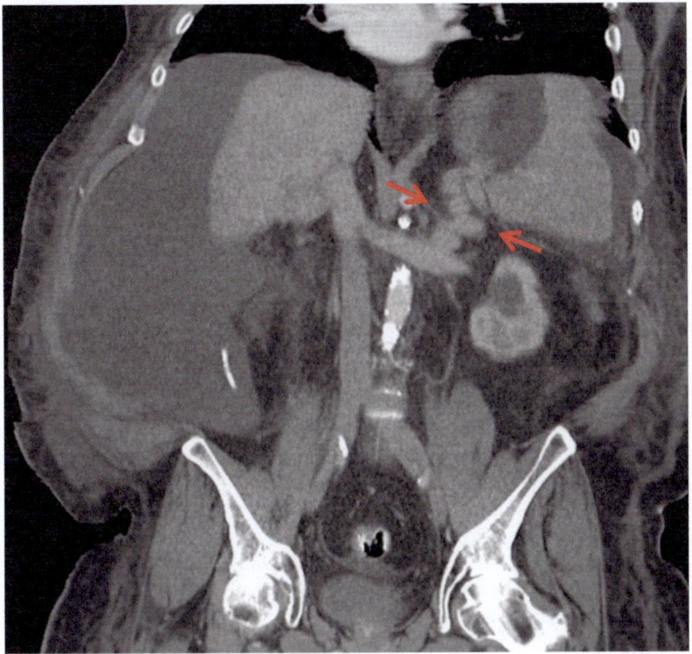

Fig. 14.1 Large spontaneous portosystemic (splenorenal) shunts. This imaging study demonstrates a large portosystemic shunt (red arrows) connecting the splenic vein and the left renal vein

Conclusions

HE is a common manifestation of end-stage liver disease and is one of the hallmarks of decompensated cirrhosis. Timely diagnosis and a balanced approach to treatment, with close involvement of patient family members and caregivers, are crucial to optimize outcomes and improve patient quality of life. Post-TIPS HE is an expected complication of this procedure and requires aggressive monitoring and treatment; similarly, refractory HE may reflect the presence of spontaneous portosystemic shunts. Once a patient with cirrhosis is diagnosed with HE, strong consideration should be given to referral for transplant evaluation.

Further Reading

1. Amodio P, Bemeur C, Butterworth R, Cordoba J, Kato A, Montagnese S, et al. The nutritional management of hepatic encephalopathy in patients with cirrhosis: International society for hepatic encephalopathy and nitrogen metabolism consensus. Hepatology. 2013;58(1):325–36. https://doi.org/10.1002/hep.26370.
2. Amodio P, Del Piccolo F, Petteno E, Mapelli D, Angeli P, Iemmolo R, et al. Prevalence and prognostic value of quantified electroencephalogram (EEG) alterations in cirrhotic patients. J Hepatol. 2001;35(1):37–45.
3. Bajaj JS. The role of microbiota in hepatic encephalopathy. Gut Microbes. 2014;5(3):397–403. https://doi.org/10.4161/gmic.28684.
4. Bajaj JS, Schubert CM, Heuman DM, Wade JB, Gibson DP, Topaz A, et al. Persistence of cognitive impairment after resolution of overt hepatic encephalopathy. Gastroenterology. 2010;138(7):2332–40. https://doi.org/10.1053/j.gastro.2010.02.015.
5. Bass NM, Mullen KD, Sanyal A, Poordad F, Neff G, Leevy CB, et al. Rifaximin treatment in hepatic encephalopathy. N Engl J Med. 2010;362(12):1071–81. https://doi.org/10.1056/NEJMoa0907893.
6. Blei AT, Cordoba J. Hepatic encephalopathy. Am J Gastroenterol. 2001;96(7):1968–76. https://doi.org/10.1111/j.1572-0241.2001.03964.x.
7. Ferenci P, Lockwood A, Mullen K, Tarter R, Weissenborn K, Blei AT. Hepatic encephalopathy–definition, nomenclature, diagnosis, and quantification: final report of the working party at the 11th World Congresses of gastroenterology, Vienna, 1998. Hepatology. 2002;35(3):716–21. https://doi.org/10.1053/jhep.2002.31250.
8. Garcia-Martinez R, Rovira A, Alonso J, Jacas C, Simon-Talero M, Chavarria L, et al. Hepatic encephalopathy is associated with post-transplant cognitive function and brain volume. Liver Transpl. 2011;17(1):38–46. https://doi.org/10.1002/lt.22197.

  9. Jones EA, Mullen KD. Theories of the pathogenesis of hepatic encephalopathy. Clin Liver Dis. 2012;16(1):7–26. https://doi.org/10.1016/j.
     cld.2011.12.010.
 10. Ortiz M, Jacas C, Cordoba J. Minimal hepatic encephalopathy:
     diagnosis, clinical significance and recommendations. J Hepatol.
     2005;42(Suppl 1):S45–53. https://doi.org/10.1016/j.jhep.2004.11.028.
 11. Saab S, Suraweera D, Au J, Saab EG, Alper TS, Tong MJ. Probiotics are
     helpful in hepatic encephalopathy: a meta-analysis of randomized trials.
     Liver Int. 2016;36(7):986–93. https://doi.org/10.1111/liv.13005.
 12. Vilstrup H, Amodio P, Bajaj J, Cordoba J, Ferenci P, Mullen KD,
     et al. Hepatic encephalopathy in chronic liver disease: 2014 practice
     guideline by the American Association for the study of liver diseases
     and the European Association for the study of the liver. Hepatology.
     2014;60(2):715–35. https://doi.org/10.1002/hep.27210.

Chapter 15
Esophageal Varices

Sofia Simona Jakab and Guadalupe Garcia-Tsao

Introduction

Variceal hemorrhage is one of the complications of cirrhosis that defines progression to the stage of decompensated cirrhosis, with a mortality as high as 40%, depending on the severity of liver disease. Therefore, it is essential to identify patients with cirrhosis at a high risk of variceal bleeding, so that prevention strategies can be implemented. In this chapter, we describe a case of a patient recently diagnosed with cirrhosis. We discuss current recommendations on screening/surveillance for esophageal varices, strategies for primary and secondary prophylaxis of esophageal variceal hemorrhage (EVH), as well as treatment options and outcomes of EVH.

S. S. Jakab · G. Garcia-Tsao (✉)
Section of Digestive Diseases, Yale University School of Medicine, New Haven, CT, USA

Section of Digestive Diseases, VA CT Healthcare System, West Haven, CT, USA
e-mail: guadalupe.garcia-tsao@yale.edu

© Springer Nature Switzerland AG 2019
S. M. Cohen, P. Davitkov (eds.), *Liver Disease*,
https://doi.org/10.1007/978-3-319-98506-0_15

Clinical Case Scenario

A 55-year-old male presents to his primary care provider after not having been seen for 10 years. He has a history of at-risk alcohol drinking, not interfering with his job as an accountant, and with no alcohol-related hospitalizations. Because of a recent motor vehicle accident (MVA) while intoxicated, he is now committed to remain sober and to reestablish medical care. He takes no medications. His physical examination is remarkable for BP 115/70, HR 75, spider angiomas, and palmar erythema. Labs done in ER post MVA showed platelet count of 90,000/ mm^3, albumin 3.3 g/dL, bilirubin 2.1 mg/dL, INR 1.4, ALT 40 U/L, and AST 120 U/L. CT of the liver revealed a nodular liver, recanalized umbilical vein, paraesophageal collaterals, and splenomegaly. His primary care provider initiates a hepatology referral for evaluation and management of cirrhosis. On presentation to the liver specialist, physical exam confirmed prior findings; in addition, he had a firm and enlarged left lobe of the liver, and palpable spleen tip; otherwise, the abdomen was not distended, and there was no shifting dullness. Transient elastography was performed and showed a liver stiffness (LS) of 25 kPa.

Questions

1. Does this patient need screening for esophageal varices?
2. What are the current screening guidelines for varices (who, how, and when to screen)?
3. Which patients with esophageal varices require primary prophylaxis of EVH? What treatments are recommended for primary prophylaxis?

4. What are the initial treatment options for a patient with suspected acute variceal bleeding?
5. What additional information should the specialist obtain at the time of suspected acute variceal bleeding?
6. What options are available to prevent recurrent variceal bleeding?

Discussion

Question 1. Does this patient need screening for esophageal varices?

This patient has cirrhosis, based on clinical (firm, enlarged left liver lobe, splenomegaly, spider angioma, palmar erythema), laboratory (thrombocytopenia, liver synthetic dysfunction with abnormal albumin, INR, bilirubin), imaging (nodular liver, portal hypertension as suggested by recanalized umbilical vein, portosystemic collaterals, splenomegaly), and elastographic findings. As he never had variceal bleeding, ascites, or hepatic encephalopathy, his cirrhosis is compensated.

CT and elastography are suggestive of clinically significant portal hypertension (defined as a hepatic venous pressure gradient of ≥ 10 mmHg), with a high likelihood of having esophageal varices, but an upper endoscopy is still necessary to assess the patient's risk for EVH, based on the presence/size of varices, and high-risk stigmata. Importantly, finding paraesophageal collaterals on imaging, while indicating the presence of clinically significant portal hypertension, does not necessarily mean that the patient has esophageal varices or that primary prophylaxis of EVH is recommended.

Question 2. What are the current screening guidelines for varices (who, how, and when to screen)?

Who

All patients with cirrhosis, either compensated or decompensated, need to be evaluated to determine the presence of varices at a high risk of bleeding (high-risk varices, HRV), which would require prophylactic therapy with nonselective beta-blockers (NSBB) or endoscopic variceal ligation (EVL).

The presence of varices depends on the severity of liver disease. Varices are present in only 30–40% of patients with Child class A cirrhosis (mostly compensated), while they are present in up to 85% of Child B and C cirrhosis (decompensated). The presence of varices in a patient with compensated cirrhosis is indicative of the presence of clinically significant portal hypertension, and it is associated with a significantly higher risk of decompensation compared to patients without varices. Therefore, screening for varices in the compensated patient is not only of clinical significance, but also of prognostic significance. The presence of varices in patients with decompensated cirrhosis, on the other hand, is associated with a higher risk of EVH and of death from EVH, particularly those belonging to Child class C.

How

Upper endoscopy (esophagogastroduodenoscopy, EGD) is the standard of care in the diagnosis and risk stratification of esophageal varices. Based on appearance on endoscopy, there are several classifications regarding the size of esophageal varices, the most commonly used being small/medium/large or only small/large. Varices that are at a high risk of bleeding are those classified as medium/large (in the 3-scale classification) or large (in the 2-scale classification).

In addition to variceal size, the presence or absence of red wale marks (areas of thinning of the variceal wall) on varices should be noted, as they are independent predictors of variceal hemorrhage.

The prevalence of high-risk varices in patients with compensated cirrhosis is very low, 10–20%. Therefore, it makes sense to pre-screen compensated patients for their likelihood of not having high-risk varices as this would circumvent invasive screening. A combination of LS, platelet count, and spleen size can identify this likelihood. The combination of LS <20 kPa *and* a platelet count above 150,000/mL is associated with a <5% chance of having high-risk varices. Therefore, it is recommended that patients with compensated cirrhosis be pre-screened using these noninvasive tests. If criteria are met, EGD could be avoided and noninvasive testing repeated on a yearly basis. In the absence of transient elastography, a stepwise approach using platelet count >150,000/mL or MELD = 6 (if platelet count <150,000/mL) may be helpful in identifying these low-risk patients, although some patients with HRV could be missed.

As patients with decompensated cirrhosis have, by definition, significant portal hypertension, screening endoscopy is recommended at the time of diagnosis in all of them, or at the time of cirrhosis decompensation (in a patient with compensated cirrhosis who develops ascites and/or hepatic encephalopathy).

When/How Often

The interval of surveillance endoscopy in compensated cirrhosis depends on specific factors associated with the risk of a more severe portal hypertension: ongoing liver injury (untreated viral hepatitis, presence of other cofactors for liver injury, i.e., obesity, alcohol), or if small varices were found on last endoscopy, or when a compensated patient develops ascites and/or hepatic encephalopathy and becomes decompensated.

In patients with compensated cirrhosis who had a screening EGD, surveillance endoscopy to detect HRV is recommended every 1–3 years:

- If there were no varices on screening endoscopy, EGD should be repeated in 2 years if ongoing liver injury, or in 3 years if inactive liver disease (normal liver enzymes) such as post-hepatitis C eradication or if alcohol abstinence.
- If there were small varices on screening endoscopy, EGD should be repeated in 1 year if ongoing liver injury, or in 2 years if inactive liver disease.

In patients with decompensated cirrhosis, surveillance endoscopy is recommended every year.

In patients with either compensated or decompensated cirrhosis in whom nonselective beta-blockers (NSBB) are chosen for primary prophylaxis (see below), there is no need for follow-up EGDs.

Recommendations regarding if and when the next endoscopy is required are outlined in Tables 15.1 and 15.2.

Table 15.1 Endoscopic surveillance of gastroesophageal varices in patients with *compensated* cirrhosis

Findings on screening EGD/most recent EGD		Next EGD will be
No varices	Inactive liver disease[a]	EGD in 3 years
	Active liver disease[b]	EGD in 2 years
Small varices without red marks[c]	Inactive liver disease	
	Active liver disease	EGD in 1 year
Small varices with red marks	Should be on NSBB	No repeat EGD
Medium/large varices	If choice is NSBB	
	If choice is EVL	EGD q2–8 weeks until eradication Once EV eradicated, EGDs q6–12 months

[a]Inactive liver disease: normal liver enzymes, treated HCV, alcohol abstinence
[b]Active liver disease: untreated HCV, alcohol use, NASH
[c]If choice to start NSBB (optional), no need to repeat EGD

Table 15.2 Endoscopic surveillance of gastroesophageal varices in patients with *decompensated* cirrhosis

Findings on screening EGD/most recent EGD		Next EGD will be
No varices	Child B or C	EGD in 1 year
Small varices without red marks[a]	Child B	EGD in 1 year
	Child C: Should be on NSBB	No repeat EGD
Small varices with red marks	Should be on NSBB	
Medium/large varices	If choice is NSBB	
	If choice is EVL	EGD q2–8 weeks until EV eradication Once EV eradicated, EGDs q6–12 months

[a]If choice to start NSBB (optional), no need to repeat EGD

Question 3. Which patients with varices require primary prophylaxis of EVH? What treatments are recommended for primary prophylaxis?

The following patients require primary prophylaxis of EVH as their risk of bleeding is >15% per year:

1. Patients with medium or large varices which constitute the largest group
2. Patients with small varices with red wale marks
3. Child C class patients with any size varices

The two therapies with a proven beneficial effect in preventing first EVH are NSBB or EVL. Either one or the other should be used, as combination therapy has no advantages and can increase side effects.

NSBBs have the advantage of decreasing portal pressure and therefore have the potential of reducing not only variceal hemorrhage but other complications of cirrhosis such as ascites. EVL is a local therapy without an effect on portal pressure and carries the risk of bleeding from ligation-induced ulcers. Additionally, EVL is not recommended in patients with high-risk small varices because small varices are difficult to ligate. Importantly, if NSBB are chosen as primary prophylactic therapy and appropriately titrated (see below, Table 15.3), there is no need for surveillance endoscopies. If EVL is chosen, endoscopy is done every 2–8 weeks if varices are large enough for band ligation; once variceal eradication is achieved, repeat endoscopy for surveillance is indicated at 3–6 months, followed by EGD every 6–12 months until large varices are detected and band ligation is required again.

Safety concerns regarding the use of NSBBs in patients with decompensated cirrhosis, particularly in patients with refractory ascites, have been raised. Earlier reports finding increased kidney dysfunction and mortality secondary to NSBBs have been challenged by subsequent studies, and it would appear that the deleterious effect is dose-dependent and related to a low mean arterial pressure. Therefore, NSBBs are not contraindicated in patients with ascites, but they require careful use: avoid high doses (not to exceed 80 mg propranolol orally twice a day or 80 mg nadolol orally daily); avoid carvedilol given its additional vasodilating effect and therefore higher likelihood to decrease blood pressure; titrate NSBBs to avoid systolic BP <90 mm Hg; and temporarily discontinue NSBBs in the setting of bleeding, infection, or kidney dysfunction.

Recommendations on therapies for primary prophylaxis of variceal bleeding are included in Table 15.3.

Additional Clinical Information

The patient underwent EGD which showed several columns of large varices, which did not flatten despite air insufflation. Nadolol was started at 20 mg daily and then titrated to 60 mg daily. On follow-up visit, his HR was 56/min, BP was 100/50,

Table 15.3 Treatment options for primary prophylaxis

Therapy	Dose	Goal
Propranolol	20–160 mg BID (if ascites, up to 80 mg BID)	Titrate to max tolerable dose or HR 55–60 or SBP <90
Nadolol	20–160 mg daily (if ascites, up to 80 mg daily)	Titrate to max tolerable dose or HR 55–60 or SBP <90
Carvedilol	3.125–12.5 mg daily (if ascites: avoid)	Titrate to 12.5 mg/day or SBP <90
EVL	EGD q2–8 weeks until EV eradication; once EV eradication, repeat EGD at 3–6 months, followed by EGD q6–12 months	Variceal eradication: resume banding q2–8 weeks if recurrent varices

and he had no side effects except for minor fatigue. A month later, he presents to the ER with hematemesis. His wife confirms alcohol abstinence and compliance with nadolol. On physical exam, BP is 85/45, HR was 110, he is alert but oriented only to self, and abdomen is distended, with shifting dullness. Laboratory studies are remarkable for Hb 8.5 g/dL (prior 13 g/dL), platelet count of 75,000/mm^3, INR 2.1, total bilirubin 2.8 mg/dL, albumin 2.5 g/dL, and creatinine 1.1 mg/dL. He was intubated in ER and admitted to MICU for possible acute variceal bleeding.

Question 4. What are the initial treatment options for a patient with suspected acute variceal bleeding?

General management of acute variceal bleeding should focus on resuscitation (i.v. access, airway/breathing/circulation), but use restrictive transfusion of packed red blood cells and start transfusion when hemoglobin is below <7 g/dL with the goal of 7–9 g/dL. Therefore, this patient does not require PRBC transfusion. There is no evidence that correcting platelet count or INR is of benefit in variceal hemorrhage. Nadolol has to be discontinued, given low blood pressure in the setting of bleeding and a potential deleterious effect of NSBB by blunting the sympathetic response to hemorrhage.

Specific pharmacologic therapy for acute variceal hemorrhage should be initiated as soon as the diagnosis is suspected and while making arrangements for an urgent upper endoscopy. This includes:

1. IV octreotide given as an initial IV bolus of 50 mcg followed by a continuous infusion of 50 mcg/h for 3 to 5 days, which will cause splanchnic vasoconstriction and a reduction in portal pressure
2. Antibiotic prophylaxis (IV ceftriaxone 1 gm/24 h), which will decrease the variceal rebleeding rate and mortality by decreasing the risk of bacterial infection (in particular spontaneous bacterial peritonitis)

Endoscopy needs to be performed within 12 h of admission, with EVL if a diagnosis of variceal hemorrhage is established based on the following criteria: (a) active bleeding from a varix, (b) stigmata of recent hemorrhage are observed on a varix (clot, white nipple), or (c) only non-bleeding varices are seen and there is no other source of bleeding.

Question 5. What additional information should the specialist obtain at the time of suspected acute variceal bleeding?

Child-Turcotte-Pugh (CTP) score, MELD score, diagnostic paracentesis, and liver ultrasound with Doppler to assess portal and hepatic vascular patency will help stratify the risk of rebleeding and mortality and help plan further treatment if necessary. A transjugular intrahepatic portosystemic shunt (TIPS) is sometimes required to treat acute variceal bleeding. TIPS is an expandable stent deployed by interventional radiology to decompress the portal venous system by creating a shunt between the portal and hepatic veins. TIPS as "rescue" therapy is usually used after 1–2 failed attempts of combined endoscopic and pharmacologic management.

In patients with a CTP score (10–13), placement of TIPS should be considered within 24–48 h from EVL as these patients are at a high risk of failing standard therapy. Placing an "early" (preemptive) TIPS prevents failure of standard therapy and reduces the mortality associated with placing a "rescue" TIPS (i.e., when it is placed after failure occurs).

For patients in whom bleeding is brisk and banding cannot be performed, balloon tamponade may help as a temporizing measure. Balloon tamponade involves using a tube with an esophageal and a gastric balloon. It requires training and following a specific protocol to avoid complications. It is effective in controlling bleeding temporarily, as a bridge to TIPS or, less likely, liver transplantation. It can cause lethal complications such as aspiration, esophageal ulceration, and perforation. Self-expandable esophageal stents have also been found to have greater efficacy and less complications than balloon tamponade in the control of EVH in treatment failures.

Question 6. What options are available to prevent recurrent variceal bleeding?

In patients who have bled from varices (and did not undergo a TIPS), the 1-year risk of recurrent VH can be as high as 60% in the absence of secondary prophylaxis. The recommended treatment to prevent recurrent hemorrhage consists of combination therapy NSBB plus EVL:

1. NSBB (nadolol or propranolol, dose and goals as per Table 15.3). In this setting, there is not enough data to recommend carvedilol as there are no randomized controlled trials, and patients may have more severe liver disease and are more prone to be more vasodilated. NSBB should be started during hospitalization, once octreotide is discontinued, to allow monitoring of BP, HR, and occurrence of any clinical side effects prior to discharge. Notably, antibiotics can be discontinued at the time octreotide is discontinued.
2. EVL every 2–8 weeks until varices are eradicated, followed by surveillance endoscopy at 3–6 months post variceal eradication, and every 6–12 months indefinitely. When large varices recur, EVL is resumed every 2–8 weeks until variceal eradication.

The key element of combination therapy is NSBB, particularly in Child B/C patients in whom a higher mortality has been shown when patients are on EVL alone compared to combination therapy NSBB + EVL.

Patients who had TIPS placed during the episode of acute EVH should not receive NSBB or EVL as the shunt resolves portal hypertension and varices. However, they will require Doppler ultrasound of the TIPS every 6 months (at the time of hepatocellular carcinoma surveillance) to assess TIPS patency.

Patient Treatment Course

Diagnostic paracentesis was negative for spontaneous bacterial peritonitis. Ultrasound Doppler showed a patent portal vein. Given CTP class C (12), the patient was referred to interventional radiology for TIPS which was successfully placed within 48 h from admission, with reduction in portosystemic gradient from

25 to 11 mm Hg. Octreotide was discontinued (once a TIPS is in place, octreotide is of no benefit, as pressure reduction achieved by TIPS is much greater than reduction with pharmacological therapy). He completed a 5-day course of IV ceftriaxone. NSBB and EVL were not recommended as the patient already had a TIPS placed, with a gradient less than 12 mm Hg (the threshold associated with complications secondary to portal hypertension). The TIPS will need evaluation with ultrasound Doppler every 6 months to check for patency. If suspicion for stenosis, he will need TIPS interrogation/revision to make sure the gradient remains less than 12 mm Hg, as in his case, recurrent variceal hemorrhage is the only clinical sign of TIPS failure.

Conclusions

Esophageal varices and variceal hemorrhage are clinical mile-stones in the natural history of cirrhosis. Specific guidelines help clinicians to screen and appropriately choose the right treatment strategy to prevent or treat variceal bleeding. Once patients have sustained a variceal hemorrhage, they should be considered for liver transplant evaluation.

Further Reading

1. Abraldes JG, Bureau C, Stefanescu H, et al. Noninvasive tools and risk of clinically significant portal hypertension and varices in compensated cirrhosis: the "anticipate" study. Hepatology. 2016;64:2173–84.
2. Albillos A, Zamora J, Martínez J, et al. Stratifying risk in the prevention of recurrent variceal hemorrhage: results of an individual patient meta-analysis. Hepatology. 2017;66(4):1219–31.

3. Conejo I, Guardascione MA, Tandon P, et al. Multicenter external validation of risk stratification criteria for patients with variceal bleeding. Clin Gastroenterol Hepatol. 2018;16(1):132–9.
4. Franchis R, Baveno VI Faculty. Expanding consensus in portal hypertension: report of the Baveno VI consensus workshop: stratifying risk and individualizing care for portal hypertension. J Hepatol. 2015;63:743–52.
5. Garcia-Tsao G, Abraldes JG, Berzigotti A, et al. Portal hypertensive bleeding in cirrhosis: risk stratification, diagnosis, and management: 2016 practice guidance by the American Association for the study of liver diseases. Hepatology. 2017;65(1):310–35.
6. Merkel C, Zoli M, Siringo S, et al. Prognostic indicators of risk for first variceal bleeding in cirrhosis: a multicenter study in 711 patients to validate and improve the North Italian Endoscopic Club (NIEC) index. Am J Gastroenterol. 2000;95(10):2915–20.
7. The European Association for the Study of the Liver. EASL clinical practice guidelines for the management of patients with decompensated cirrhosis. J Hepatol. 2018;69(2):406–60.

Chapter 16
Autoimmune Hepatitis

John F. Reinus and Kristina R. Chacko

Introduction

Autoimmune hepatitis (AIH) is a chronic inflammatory liver disease with a wide range of clinical manifestations. Affected individuals may be asymptomatic with mildly elevated serum aminotransferase levels or may present with acute liver failure. While most common in young women, the disease can occur in men and women of all ages and ethnicities. AIH is the result of a complex interaction of environmental triggers, genetic predisposition, and failure of immune tolerance. Immunosuppression with corticosteroids and other immunomodulator therapies are

J. F. Reinus · K. R. Chacko (✉)
Division of Gastroenterology and Liver Diseases,
Department of Medicine, Montefiore Medical Center,
Albert Einstein College of Medicine, Bronx, NY, USA
e-mail: krchacko@montefiore.org

© Springer Nature Switzerland AG 2019
S. M. Cohen, P. Davitkov (eds.), *Liver Disease*,
https://doi.org/10.1007/978-3-319-98506-0_16

the cornerstones of treatment. Left untreated, AIH can progress to cirrhosis and is the underlying reason for up to 5% of liver transplants.

Clinical Case Scenario

A 26-year-old black female presents for complaints of several months of fatigue and malaise. She has no prior medical history, including immune-mediated disease. Her only medication is an oral contraceptive, which she has taken daily for 8 years; she does not take herbal supplements and has no history of drug use. She drinks one to two glasses of wine on the weekends. There is no family history of liver disease, although her mother and sister have hypothyroidism and her father has diabetes. Her physical exam is remarkable for a BMI of 29 and anicteric conjunctivae. She has no stigmata of chronic liver disease, including no spider angioma or palmar erythema. Notable lab test results are ALT 393 U/L, AST 355 U/L, alkaline phosphatase 136 U/L, and total bilirubin 1.2 mg/dL. She was seen by her PCP 6 weeks ago, and at that time, her ALT and AST levels were 251 U/L and 145 U/L, respectively. Her CBC and basic metabolic panel are normal. She is referred to a hepatologist for further evaluation of the elevated liver enzymes.

Questions

1. What is the differential diagnosis of this patient's abnormal liver enzyme levels?
2. What are the criteria for diagnosis of AIH?
3. What is the natural history of AIH?
4. What are the treatment options for this patient?
5. What is the appropriate management strategy of AIH in pregnancy?

Discussion

Question 1. What is the differential diagnosis of this patient's abnormal liver enzyme levels?

This young woman has a moderate-severe elevation of her serum aminotransferase levels (>10× ULN) and mild elevation of her total bilirubin and alkaline phosphatase levels, characterized as a predominantly hepatocellular pattern. Given the persistent abnormality of the serum aminotransferase results over a period of 6 weeks, she warrants an evaluation for possible chronic liver disease. The differential diagnosis is quite broad, including viral, autoimmune, fatty, and metabolic liver diseases. She is not on any medications or supplements that cause hepatitis, nor does she drink excessive amounts of alcohol or have risk factors for infection with parenterally transmitted hepatitis viruses. Her BMI is 29, and she has a family history of diabetes, which is associated with the development of non-alcoholic fatty liver disease (NAFLD), although her AST and ALT are higher than is typically seen with fatty liver disease. Other less common metabolic diseases, such as Wilson's disease and hereditary hemochromatosis, can be considered and screened with a serum ceruloplasmin test and iron studies. Autoimmune diseases, including AIH, primary biliary cholangitis (PBC, formerly "primary biliary cirrhosis"), and primary sclerosing cholangitis (PSC), also need to be considered. Autoantibodies used to diagnose autoimmune liver diseases are shown in Table 16.1.

Additional Clinical Information

In order to make a definitive diagnosis, she requires further blood tests, imaging, and potentially a liver biopsy. Viral serologies for hepatitis B and C show she is immune to hepatitis B and has never been exposed to hepatitis C. The results of iron studies

Table 16.1 Autoantibodies in the diagnosis of autoimmune hepatitis

Antibody	Target antigen	Liver disease
ANA	Multiple targets Chromatin Ribonucleoproteins	AIH PBC PSC Drug-induced NAFLD HBV/HCV
SMA	Microfilaments (f-actin)	Same as ANA
LKM1	Cytochrome p450	Type 2 AIH HCV
LC1		Type 2 AIH
pANCA	Nuclear lamina proteins	Type 1 AIH PSC
AMA	E2-subunit of pyruvate dehydrogenase	AIH PBC

and ceruloplasmin level are normal. Her abdominal ultrasound shows a liver that is normal in size and echogenicity. Autoimmune serologies are ordered, including antinuclear antibodies (ANA), anti-smooth muscle antibody (SMA), anti-liver-kidney-microsomal antibody (LKM1), and anti-mitochondrial antibody (AMA). The results are ANA-positive (1:160) and SMA-positive (1:40). LKM1 and AMA tests are negative. The serum IgG level is abnormal (2400 mg/dL); IgM and IgA levels are normal. She undergoes an ultrasound-guided liver biopsy for diagnosis.

Question 2. What are the criteria for diagnosis of AIH?

Given their variable clinical presentations, autoimmune liver diseases are often challenging to diagnose. This is especially true when patients are asymptomatic or have an insidious disease onset. To facilitate diagnosis, the International Autoimmune Hepatitis Group has developed a scoring system that incorporates a number of clinical and laboratory features (Table 16.2). Based

Table 16.2 Revised original scoring system of the International Autoimmune Hepatitis Group

Sex	Female	+2	**ANA, SMA, LKM-1**	>1:80	+3
AP/AST ratio	<1.5	+2		1:80	+2
	1.5–3.0	0		1:40	+1
	>3.0	−2		<1:40	0
IgG	>2.0	+3	**AMA positive**		−4
	1.5–2.0	+2	**Viral markers**	Positive	−3
	1.0–1.5	+1	**Alcohol intake**	<25 g/d	+2
	<1.0	0		>60 g/d	−2
Histology	Interface hepatitis	+3			
	Lymphoplasmacytic infiltrate	+1			
	Rosettes	+1	Biliary changes		−3
	None of the above	−5	Other features		−3
Response to treatment	Complete	+2			
	Relapse	+3			

Interpretation

Pretreatment			**Posttreatment**		
Definite AIH		>15	Definite AIH		>17
Probable AIH		10–15	Probable AIH		12–17

on this scoring system, patients may be classified as "definite" or "probable" AIH with additional points assigned based on response to treatment. Histology remains the key element in making the diagnosis of AIH.

Laboratory findings in AIH may vary widely, ranging from mild (3–5× ULN) to severe (>50× ULN) elevations of the serum aminotransferase levels, typically in a hepatocellular pattern. It is important to recognize that the degree of ALT elevation does not always reflect the histological severity of disease, and these levels may fluctuate spontaneously, even normalizing, despite ongoing histologic inflammation. Elevated IgG levels are present in approximately 85% of individuals with AIH. The range of "normal" gamma globulin levels is wide, and patients may have a relatively elevated IgG level that is still within the normal range and that decreases significantly with medical therapy. Despite these limitations, normalization of the aminotransferase and IgG levels is considered the marker of biochemical remission.

Serologic testing for antibodies remains a key part of the diagnosis of AIH (Table 16.1). In North America, 96% of affected patients will have a positive ANA, SMA, or both (AIH Type 1), and 4% will have LKM1 or LC1 (AIH Type 2). LKM1 antibodies are more common in European patients with AIH. Despite their importance, autoantibody titers may fluctuate during the disease course, and patients who are seronegative at initial presentation may have positive serologies later. Individuals presenting with severe or fulminant disease are more likely than those with mild to moderate disease to be seronegative.

Liver biopsy is necessary to establish the diagnosis of AIH and guide treatment. The histologic hallmark of AIH is interface hepatitis: a lymphoplasmacytic infiltrate at the limiting plate of the portal tract. Other characteristic features include hepatocellular rosette formation, lobular hepatitis with a predominance of plasma cells, and hepatocyte swelling. In severe acute AIH or acute liver failure, extensive necrosis and pan-lobular hepatitis with parenchymal collapse may occur. The presence of granulomas, steatosis, and bile duct damage may suggest an alternative diagnosis. In addition to providing diagnostic information, the extent of fibrosis and necrosis can affect management, including timing of immunosuppressive treatment and even the potential need for consideration of liver transplantation.

Additional Clinical Information

The patient's liver biopsy shows moderate to severe interface hepatitis with lymphoplasmacytic infiltrates and stage 2 (of 4) fibrosis. The findings are consistent with AIH.

Question 3. What is the natural history of AIH?

Approximately 25% of patients with AIH will initially present with severe acute hepatitis and even liver failure, and a significant portion of these individuals will have hepatic fibrosis or cirrhosis. Black patients have a more aggressive disease course and are more likely to present with acute liver failure and cirrhosis as compared to non-black patients. Additionally, they are less likely to respond to immunosuppression and have an overall poorer outcome.

One-third of AIH patients will present with non-specific symptoms, such as fatigue, malaise, anorexia, weight loss, nausea, pruritus, and jaundice. Patients may have stigmata of chronic liver disease, including palmar erythema, hepatosplenomegaly, and manifestations of portal hypertension. Approximately 35–45% of patients will be asymptomatic at initial diagnosis, something more commonly seen in men and persons with lower serum aminotransferase levels. Despite the absence of symptoms, up to one-third of these patients will have cirrhosis, suggesting that they have had subclinical disease for a long time. The presence of cirrhosis at diagnosis is most common in younger (<20 years) or older (>60 years) patients.

Spontaneous remission of AIH is rare, so while patients with mild or no symptoms have a good prognosis, they require close monitoring and early consideration for treatment. AIH is a progressive disease and may evolve rapidly with early development of cirrhosis and death if left untreated. Predictors of a poor outcome include the absence of normalization of ALT after 6 months, younger (<20 years) or older (>60 years) age at presentation, and black race. The risk of hepatocellular carcinoma (HCC) is lower in AIH than it is in other forms of chronic liver disease, but HCC can occur in AIH patients with cirrhosis.

Question 4. What are the treatment options for this patient?

The goal of treatment in AIH is to prevent progression of disease and need for liver transplantation while minimizing the adverse effects of immunosuppression. Successful treatment is characterized by both biochemical and histological remission, which is defined as the normalization of serum aminotransferase levels and the absence of portal inflammation and interface hepatitis on liver biopsy. Given the potential adverse effects of immunosuppressive therapy, some experts favor monitoring individuals with mild or inactive disease, or contraindications to therapy, with frequent liver tests and IgG levels. Patients with symptoms or active inflammation on biopsy should be treated. The American Association for the Study of Liver Diseases (AASLD) treatment recommendations are summarized in Table 16.3.

Table 16.3 AASLD indications for immunosuppressive treatment

Absolute	Relative	None
AST >10× ULN	Symptoms of fatigue, arthralgia, jaundice	Asymptomatic with normal AST and globulins
AST >5× ULN and globulin >2× ULN	AST 2–5× ULN and globulins 1–2× ULN	Inactive cirrhosis, mild portal inflammation
Bridging or multiacinar necrosis	Interface hepatitis	Severe cytopenia, TPMT deficiency
Incapacitating symptoms	Osteopenia, emotional instability, hypertension, diabetes, cytopenia	Pathologic fractures, psychosis, uncontrolled diabetes, or hypertension

The initial treatment for patients with AIH may be prednisone alone or in combination with azathioprine. In patients receiving prednisone monotherapy, the initial dose is up to 60 mg/day and is tapered slowly to 20 mg daily over 4 weeks. To reduce steroid-associated side effects such as moon facies, acne, hirsutism, diabetes, and weight gain, combination therapy with prednisone 30 mg/day and weight-based azathioprine (1–2 mg/kg/day) is preferred by many practitioners. Prednisone is tapered slowly, and maintenance treatment is continued with azathioprine alone or with prednisone 5 mg daily. Ninety percent of patients will have biochemical evidence of response within 2 weeks, while histologic improvement may take 3 to 8 months. Treatment should be continued for at least 2 years after biochemical remission, and a liver biopsy is recommended in order to confirm histologic improvement before terminating treatment. This should be done with caution as 80% of patients who have had biochemical and histological remission will relapse after stopping therapy. Multiple relapses have been associated with higher rates of cirrhosis, liver failure, and liver transplantation. For this reason, long-term maintenance therapy with azathioprine is recommended.

Budesonide, a synthetic glucocorticoid with a 90% hepatic first pass metabolism, may be used in place of prednisone as the initial treatment of AIH. The low systemic bioavailability of budesonide may protect patients from developing steroid-associated side effects. Recent studies have shown that budesonide may be used as first-line therapy in combination with azathioprine in non-cirrhotic patients.

In patients who fail treatment despite adherence, the doses of prednisone and azathioprine may be increased. For those patients who don't respond to first-line treatment, alternative regimens that include mycophenolate mofetil or calcineurin antagonists, such as cyclosporine or tacrolimus, may be tried.

Patients with decompensated AIH cirrhosis or acute liver failure should be evaluated quickly for liver transplantation. End-stage liver disease and liver failure due to AIH is the indication for approximately 5% of liver transplants performed in the USA. Survival after liver transplantation for patients with AIH is excellent: 5- and 10-year survivals are approximately 75% as compared to less than 30% in untreated patients. While immune-mediated hepatitis after transplantation for AIH occurs in as many as 30% of recipients, treatment with increased immunosuppressive therapy can successfully prevent graft loss in most cases.

Additional Clinical Information

The patient begins treatment with prednisone 30 mg and azathioprine 50 mg daily and is educated regarding the possible adverse effects of treatment with these drugs (bone marrow suppression, infection, pancreatitis, lymphoma, hypertension, hyperglycemia, weight gain, and osteoporosis). Screening for latent infections including tuberculosis and hepatitis B is performed before initiating therapy. Laboratory studies at treatment week 4 include an ALT level of 43 U/L and an IgG level of 1900 mg/dL. Based on her weight of 80 kg, her azathioprine dose is increased to 100 mg daily, and her dose of prednisone is tapered slowly over the next 6 weeks, with normalization of her liver enzyme and IgG levels.

She remains in remission over the next 3 years on maintenance therapy with azathioprine 100 mg daily and then returns to your office reporting that she is getting married and is planning to start a family. She inquires about the risk of stopping her immunosuppressive treatment during and after pregnancy.

Question 5. What is the appropriate management of AIH in pregnancy?

There is an increased risk of pregnancy-related complications for women with AIH. Published reports have found that the risk of fetal loss is 25% and preterm birth up to 15%. While remission of disease may occur during the second and third trimesters, flares of disease, including acute liver failure, have been reported following delivery.

There is a growing body of data on treatment with azathioprine during pregnancy. Despite a category D classification by the FDA, studies of patients with inflammatory bowel disease or AIH have shown therapy with azathioprine during pregnancy is safe. The use of this drug has not been associated with increased rates of fetal complications. In patients in whom therapy has been discontinued, higher rates of maternal complications related to disease flare or decompensation have been found. For this reason, continued maintenance therapy with azathioprine or prednisone, or both, during and after pregnancy is recommended. Patients treated with mycophenolate mofetil, which is teratogenic, must continue to use contraception until they are transitioned to an alternative form of treatment.

Conclusions

The clinical presentation of AIH varies widely. Patients who may have AIH require a thorough diagnostic evaluation, including autoimmune serologies, liver tests, and liver biopsy. While the presentation of AIH may be acute, a large portion of affected patients already will have significant fibrosis and even cirrhosis at the time of diagnosis. A variety of factors, including genetics, race, and age at disease onset all have important prognostic implications. Immunosuppressive therapy in patients with active disease can successfully prevent disease progression.

Further Reading

1. Alvarez F, Berg PA, Bianchi FB, et al. International Autoimmune Hepatitis Group Report: Review of criteria for diagnosis of autoimmune hepatitis. J Hepatol. 1999;31:929–39.

2. European Association for the Study of the Liver. EASL clinical practice guidelines: autoimmune hepatitis. J Hepatol. 2015;63(4):971.
3. Feld JJ, Dinh H, Arenovich T, Marcus VA, Wanless IR, Heathcote EJ. Autoimmune hepatitis: effect of symptoms and cirrhosis on natural history and outcome. Hepatology. 2005;42(1):53–62.
4. Manns MP, Czaja AJ, Gorham JD, Krawitt EL, Mieli-Vergani G, Vergani D, Vierling JM. Diagnosis and management of autoimmune hepatitis. Hepatology. 2010;51(6):2193–213.
5. Manns MP, Jaeckel E, Taubert R. Budesonide in autoimmune hepatitis: the right drug at the right time for the right patient. Clin Gastroenterol Hepatol. 2018;16(2):186–9.
6. Ngu JH, Gearry RB, Frampton CM, Stedman CA. Predictors of poor outcome in patients with autoimmune hepatitis: a population-based study. Hepatology. 2013;57(6):2399–406.
7. Schramm C, Herkel J, Beuers U, Kanzler S, Galle PR, Lohse AW. Pregnancy in autoimmune hepatitis: outcome and risk factors. Am J Gastroenterol. 2006;101(3):556.
8. Verma S, Torbenson M, Thuluvath PJ. The impact of ethnicity on the natural history of autoimmune hepatitis. Hepatology. 2007;46(6):1828–35.

Chapter 17
Primary Biliary Cholangitis

Andrew R. Scheinberg and Cynthia Levy

Introduction

Primary biliary cholangitis (PBC), previously known as primary biliary cirrhosis, is the most common autoimmune liver disease. PBC is characterized as a chronic inflammatory autoimmune cholestatic liver disease where immune-mediated injury to biliary epithelial cells leads to cholestasis and fibrosis, and if left untreated, PBC will progress to end-stage liver disease. The disease affects predominantly middle-aged women, with data suggesting 1 in 1000 women over the age of 40 live with PBC. Importantly, clinical presentation ranges from being completely asymptomatic to significantly affecting the patient's quality of life via pruritus, fatigue, abdominal pain, and sicca symptoms (dry mouth, dry eyes) in addition to liver-related complications. In this chapter, we describe the classic presentation of an asymptomatic patient with a cholestatic pattern of liver injury.

A. R. Scheinberg
Department of Internal Medicine, University of Miami Miller School
of Medicine/Jackson Memorial Hospital, Miami, FL, USA

C. Levy (✉)
Division of Hepatology, University of Miami Miller School
of Medicine, Miami, FL, USA
e-mail: clevy@med.miami.edu

© Springer Nature Switzerland AG 2019

S. M. Cohen, P. Davitkov (eds.), *Liver Disease*,
https://doi.org/10.1007/978-3-319-98506-0_17

We discuss the initial work-up and differential diagnosis for this pattern, the diagnostic criteria for PBC, and specific treatment, with an emphasis on early referral to a liver specialist to ensure the proper management of this progressive liver disease.

Clinical Case Scenario

A 48-year-old Hispanic woman with medical history significant for hypertension and GERD presents to her primary care provider for a routine physical examination. She feels well with no complaints and denies any gastrointestinal symptoms. Past surgical history is significant for uncomplicated cesarean section about 20 years ago. Her only medication is as needed antacids, and she denies the use of any over-the-counter medication or herbal supplements. She denies any allergies. Family history is unremarkable for gastrointestinal or liver disease. She is married with one healthy son and currently works as a school teacher. She denies tobacco use, drinks alcohol on special occasions, and denies any history of illicit drug use including IV drugs. She has never received a blood transfusion or had any tattoos. Her physical examination is unremarkable except for her liver edge being palpable below her costal margin. She exhibits no signs of chronic liver disease. Routine bloodwork shows normal blood counts, kidney function, and electrolytes. Her alkaline phosphatase (ALP) is significantly elevated at 450 IU/L (normal 44–147 IU/L). The remainder of her liver chemistries is normal.

Questions

1. What are the next steps in the evaluation of an elevated alkaline phosphatase?

2. Once confirmed to be of hepatic origin, what is the differential diagnosis of a cholestatic pattern of liver injury? What is the next step in our work-up?
3. What are the diagnostic criteria of PBC?
4. What are the treatment options for a patient with PBC?
5. What are some ways to estimate prognosis of a patient with PBC?
6. What are the other important considerations in the management of a patient with PBC?

Discussion

Question 1. What is the next step in the evaluation of an elevated alkaline phosphatase?

The finding of an elevated ALP in an asymptomatic patient requires investigation. Importantly, ALP is not only of hepatic origin as it is also found in bone, placenta, intestine, and kidney, with the most common extrahepatic location being the bone. Table 17.1 outlines specific non-hepatic etiologies for an elevated ALP.

Table 17.1 Non-hepatic causes of an elevated alkaline phosphatase

Bone disease
Osteomalacia
Paget disease
Vitamin D deficiency
Primary bone malignancy
Childhood growth
Chronic renal failure
Congestive heart failure
Lymphoma
Pregnancy

The next step in confirming that an elevated ALP is of hepatobiliary origin is measurement of the gamma-glutamyltranspeptidase (GGT). Per the American College of Gastroenterology's 2017 clinical guidelines, GGT should not be used as a screening test for underlying liver disease in the absence of abnormal liver chemistries. On the other hand, in the presence of an abnormal AST or ALT, confirmation with GGT is not necessary as the elevated alkaline phosphatase level is most likely of hepatic origin. 5-nucleotidase (5NT) is also a marker for hepatobiliary origin of an elevated ALP and is more specific than GGT; however, a normal 5NT level does not exclude a hepatic origin for an elevated ALP. Fractionation of ALP isoenzymes can be done to ascertain the origin of an elevated ALP. However, results are often unhelpful, and thus this is not routinely recommended.

Question 2. Once confirmed to be of hepatobiliary origin, what is the differential diagnosis of a cholestatic pattern of liver injury? What are the next steps in our work-up?

The differential diagnosis of a cholestatic pattern of liver injury is broad and requires a thorough history, extensive bloodwork, and radiologic imaging. The differential diagnosis of extrahepatic versus intrahepatic cholestasis is outlined in Table 17.2. Specific questions should be targeted toward gastrointestinal symptoms that may be linked to the presence of cholelithiasis, the presence of any family history significant for hepatic or biliary disease, vaccination status against viral hepatitis, sexual history, travel history, smoking and alcohol use, current or formerly used medications, and the use of herbal supplements. Multiple medications have been linked to cholestatic liver injury including phenytoin, amoxicillin/clavulanic acid, trimethoprim/sulfamethoxazole, anabolic steroids, and azathioprine. It is well-known that herbal supplements, which are not regulated by

Table 17.2 Extrahepatic and intrahepatic etiologies of a cholestatic pattern of liver injury

Extrahepatic
AIDS cholangiopathy
Bile duct obstruction
Choledocholithiasis
Malignant obstruction
Bile duct hepatobiliary flukes
Bile duct stricture
Cholestatic liver diseases
IgG4-associated cholangitis
Primary sclerosing cholangitis
Secondary sclerosing cholangitis due to cholangiolithiasis, ischemia, vasculitis
Cystic fibrosis
Intrahepatic
Primary biliary cholangitis
Primary sclerosing cholangitis
Alcoholic and nonalcoholic steatohepatitis
Cirrhosis from any etiology
Drug-induced liver injury
Graft-versus-host disease
Infiltrative diseases of the liver
Amyloidosis
Lymphoma
Sarcoidosis
Tuberculosis
Paraneoplastic syndromes, such as in Hodgkin's disease, renal cell carcinoma
Intrahepatic cholestasis of pregnancy
Genetic disorders: BRIC, PFIC, ABCB4 deficiency
Erythropoietic protoporphyria
Hepatocellular carcinoma
Nodular regenerative hyperplasia
Sepsis
Total parenteral nutrition
Vascular disease, e.g., Budd-Chiari syndrome, sinusoidal obstruction syndrome
Viral hepatitis

the FDA, are also linked to liver injury and these include green tea, chaparral leaf, germander, kava, mistletoe, toxic alkaloids, and pennyroyal.

The next step in evaluation of this patient is an abdominal ultrasound. This sensitive, noninvasive, and relatively inexpensive test is essential to differentiate between intrahepatic and extrahepatic processes and can exclude mechanical bile duct obstruction, mass lesions, and gallbladder pathology. Notably, while an abdominal ultrasound is the best imaging technique, it also has its limitations, especially the fact that it is operator-dependent. Furthermore, biliary duct dilatation may not be observed. In the setting of an elevated ALP of hepatobiliary origin and a normal abdominal ultrasound, a diagnosis of intrahepatic cholestasis is highly likely.

Back to our patient, she returns to her primary care physician about 6 months later. She now complains of some fatigue, but her physical exam remains unremarkable. She undergoes further blood work which shows her ALP is now 523 U/L, her AST is 36 IU/L, ALT 41 IU/L, and her total bilirubin is 1.0 mg/dL. Her GGT is also elevated, further confirming that her elevated ALP is of hepatobiliary origin. She is HIV negative. Her viral hepatitis panel indicates she is not immune to hepatitis A, immune to hepatitis B via vaccination, and negative for hepatitis C. Next, her primary care physician appropriately orders an abdominal ultrasound which shows no intra- or extrahepatic masses, no biliary duct dilatation, and no abnormalities of the gallbladder.

To summarize, our patient is a middle-aged woman with no significant medical history, who has complaints of fatigue with an unremarkable physical exam, found to have blood work showing a cholestatic pattern of liver injury and an unremarkable abdominal ultrasound. This is concerning for intrahepatic cholestasis.

At this juncture in time, the next step in our evaluation is geared toward evaluating for causes of intrahepatic cholestasis. This includes testing for anti-mitochondrial antibody (AMA), anti-smooth muscle antibody (ASMA), antinuclear antibodies (ANA), and anticentromere antibody. It is relevant to mention that AMA is highly specific for PBC, and while there are false-positives, it is the serological hallmark test for diagnosing PBC. In this scenario, if the AMA is negative and ANA is positive, it is worth testing for PBC-specific ANAs such as anti-gp210 and anti-sp100, when available.

In some cases, in the setting of a normal abdominal ultrasound with high suspicion for intra- or extrahepatic biliary pathology, a magnetic resonance cholangiopancreatography (MRCP) may be used to further evaluate the biliary tree. Lastly, when the work-up thus far is unrevealing, a liver biopsy should be performed for clarification.

Our patient's PCP orders the appropriate serological markers for a cholestatic pattern of liver injury. Her bloodwork reveals a persistently elevated ALP, a negative ASMA, and a positive AMA, raising concern for a diagnosis of PBC. Due to the progressive nature of PBC without treatment leading to end-stage liver disease, it is imperative to emphasize and advocate for early referral to a gastroenterologist or liver specialist.

Question 3. What are the diagnostic criteria of primary biliary cholangitis?

PBC should be suspected in patients with chronic cholestatic patterns in their bloodwork and/or symptoms of cholestasis such as fatigue and pruritus. The hallmark serological test for PBC is the presence of the AMA, observed in more than 90% of patients. While a positive AMA in the setting of a normal ALP is not diagnostic of PBC, these patients should be re-evaluated annually for the development of cholestasis.

According to the American Association for the Study of Liver Diseases (AASLD) and the European Association for the Study of the Liver (EASL) guidelines, the diagnosis of PBC can be established with the presence of two of the following criteria: (1) an elevated ALP >1.5 times the upper limit of normal, (2) the presence of AMA at a titer $\geq$1:40, and (3) liver biopsy showing non-suppurative destructive cholangitis and destruction of small- and medium-sized interlobular bile ducts.

For those patients who are AMA negative, a diagnosis of PBC can be established in the presence of PBC-specific ANA antibodies such as anti-sp100 or anti-gp210. Usually, a liver biopsy is not necessary for the diagnosis unless PBC-specific antibodies are absent, and coexistent autoimmune hepatitis (AIH) or non-alcoholic steatohepatitis (NASH) is suspected. The coexistence of PBC and AIH, known as "the overlap syndrome," is a complex diagnosis and beyond the scope of this chapter; however, it is important to mention that the presence of autoantibodies such as ANA and ASMA, a simultaneous mild elevation in the transaminases, and mild interface hepatitis on histology are commonly found in PBC and do not automatically signify the coexistence of AIH.

According to the AASLD guidelines, based on a persistent cholestatic pattern of liver injury in the presence of a positive AMA, our patient is diagnosed with PBC.

Question 4. What are the treatment options of a patient with primary biliary cholangitis?

PBC is a chronic slowly progressing disorder; however, the consequences of not treating may ultimately lead to end-stage liver disease and the need for liver transplant. Untreated PBC patients have estimated survival rates of 65% at 7 years and 60% at 10 years.

First-line treatment of PBC consists of UDCA, based on a combined analysis of three large randomized controlled trials showing improved survival for patients on UDCA when compared to those on placebo. Current guidelines recommend UDCA be dosed at 13–15 mg/kg per day as either a single daily dose or divided doses. UDCA is very well tolerated, and its side effect profile is minimal; however, at times, patients may report abdominal discomfort, constipation or diarrhea, hair thinning, or weight gain during the first year of use. Furthermore, UDCA is not believed to be teratogenic and is considered safe during pregnancy and while breastfeeding. Studies have shown UDCA markedly improves liver enzymes, slows progression of fibrosis, delays development of esophageal varices, and is linked to longer transplant-free survival time. For these reasons, AASLD and EASL recommend lifelong UDCA use as first-line pharmacotherapy.

Despite UDCA's proven efficacy in treating PBC, about 30–50% of patients do not adequately respond to UDCA. Recently, a new drug was added to the treatment repertoire for PBC, obeticholic acid (OCA). Patients who continue to have an elevated level of their ALP >1.5× ULN despite being on optimal doses of UDCA for more than 1 year or those that cannot tolerate UDCA can be started on OCA at 5 mg daily. This dose should be titrated to 10 mg daily at 3–6 months if marked improvement or normalization of ALP is not observed and if the patient is tolerating the medication well. Importantly, OCA is not recommended in patients with decompensated cirrhosis, specifically Child-Pugh B or C, due to the possibility of causing worsening liver disease and death. While OCA's side effect profile is minimal, it is associated with a dose-dependent exacerbation in pruritus which may limit its use. For this reason, it is important to simultaneously manage the symptoms associated with PBC as we will discuss later. OCA also affects serum lipids, causing a decrease in HDL cholesterol and a mild increase in LDL cholesterol. Therefore, one should monitor the patient's lipid profile and initiate statin therapy when indicated.

In addition to UDCA and OCA, other treatment modalities such as budesonide and fibrates have been examined. Based on the data from limited trials, the use of budesonide is mostly restricted to patients with overlapping features of PBC and AIH, and its use should be avoided in cirrhotic patients due to increased risk of developing portal vein thrombosis. Fibrates are well-known for their potent anti-cholestatic effects and are under investigation for use in PBC.

Question 5. What are some ways to estimate prognosis of a patient with primary biliary cholangitis?

Due to the progressive nature of PBC, it is essential to monitor every patient for adequate response to treatment and prevent the progression to end-stage liver disease. Many research trials have examined factors that affect the prognosis of patients with PBC. Established factors associated with a poor prognosis include younger age at presentation (less than 45 years), male gender, and Hispanic ethnicity. Notably, men usually present at a later age with more advanced disease and have a poorer response to UDCA. Regarding serological markers, total bilirubin and ALP are major predictors of outcome and are readily available in clinical practice. Moreover, the aspartate aminotransferase-to-platelet ratio index (APRI) score may be used to predict the presence of fibrosis and progression to cirrhosis. An APRI score greater than 0.7 and 1.0 suggests the presence of hepatic fibrosis and cirrhosis, respectively, and correlates with worse transplant-free time and overall survival time.

Vibration-controlled transient elastography (VCTE) can effectively assess liver stiffness measurement (LSM) and noninvasively detect severe fibrosis or cirrhosis. Current literature shows values of liver stiffness greater than 9.6 kPa are associated with a fivefold increase risk of liver decompensation, liver transplantation, or death, and moreover worsening LSMs over time may indicate progression of PBC. If available, the routine use of VCTE to establish stage of disease at baseline and during follow-up is recommended. It is worthwhile to mention that while liver biopsy is not routinely recommended in the management of PBC, there are various histological findings associated with a poorer prognosis.

As mentioned earlier, one must routinely evaluate PBC patients for response to UDCA. There are a multitude of definitions used to determine response to UDCA. Most definitions evaluate response at the 12-month mark from UDCA initiation and typically examine the two most important prognostic parameters, ALP and total bilirubin. The Globe PBC scoring system is now recommended by EASL to better define the individual risk of requiring liver transplant or suffering death. This model includes assessment of age at presentation, bilirubin, ALP, albumin, and platelet count at 12 months from UDCA initiation and is available online (globalpbc.com). A risk score >0.3 indicates decreased survival free of liver transplantation. In general terms, a patient with an ALP <1.5× ULN and a normal total bilirubin after 1 year of treatment with UDCA has similar transplant-free survival compared to a healthy control.

In summary, current guidelines recommend the use of VCTE, if available, in combination with the GLOBE score to help evaluate prognosis and define the risk of developing complications of advanced liver disease.

Back to our patient, she returns to your office 1 year after starting UDCA for follow-up. She reports her fatigue is improved, and she denies any pruritus or other symptoms of PBC. She is also tolerating her UDCA.

Her most recent blood work reveals AST 31 IU/L, ALT 34 IU/L, ALP 150 U/L, bilirubin 0.9 mg/dL, albumin 3.8 gm/dL, and platelets 212,000. Her transient elastography shows a liver stiffness of 5.5 kPa, indicating minimal fibrosis.

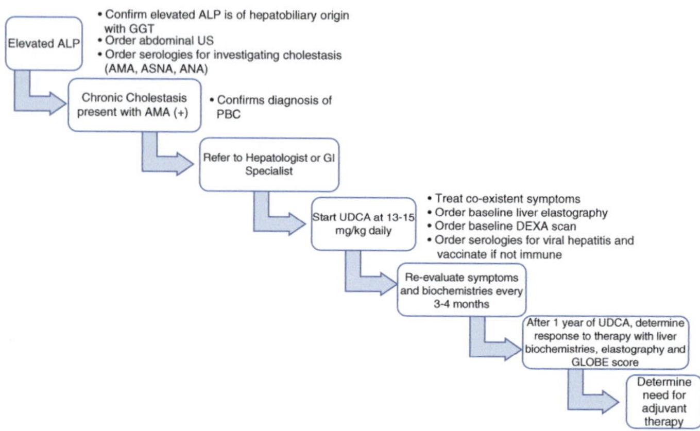

Fig. 17.1 Evaluation and treatment algorithm for primary biliary cholangitis

After reviewing her bloodwork, GLOBE score, and elastography, you explain to her that she has responded extremely well to UDCA and, if she continues on this trajectory, she should have a similar prognosis as a healthy control.

Figure 17.1 summarizes the evaluation and treatment algorithm of PBC patients

Question 6. What are the other important considerations in the management of a patient with PBC?

PBC can be associated with significant symptoms including pruritus, fatigue, and sicca symptoms (dry mouth, dry eyes). The clinician must continuously evaluate every patient for the presence of symptoms and offer effective treatment as they have a negative impact on quality of life. Since there is no correlation between disease stage and these symptoms, patients may have normal liver enzymes, minimal inflammation or fibrosis, and still be symptomatic.

Pruritus is a common symptom of cholestatic liver disease. Specific treatments used for the management of pruritus include bile acid sequestrants, most commonly cholestyramine. Patients should be instructed to take bile acid sequestrants at least a couple of hours apart from their UDCA and/or OCA as the resin interferes with bile acid (UDCA, OCA) absorption. A second-line agent for pruritus is rifampicin; however, its use has been limited by an increased risk of hepatotoxicity, which occurs in up to 10% of patients. Naltrexone, an opioid antagonist, and the selective serotonin reuptake inhibitors (SSRIs) such as sertraline have also been shown to be effective for cholestatic pruritus. For refractory itching, plasmapheresis has shown some effectiveness. In some extreme cases, refractory itching can be an indication for liver transplantation.

Fatigue is commonly reported among patients with PBC and is a significant cause of poor quality of life. Moreover, fatigue associated with PBC may be difficult to manage. Other causes of fatigue such as hypothyroidism, anemia, adrenal insufficiency, depression, and sleep disturbances should be ruled out. Counseling your patient on avoiding social isolation, engaging in coping strategies, and seeking social support is also critical to managing PBC-associated fatigue.

Sicca complex (dry mouth, dry eyes) is also frequently observed in the patient with PBC, and artificial tears and saliva are helpful in managing these symptoms. Refractory symptoms may require specialist management.

Extrahepatic complications of PBC include osteoporosis, fat-soluble vitamin deficiencies, and hyperlipidemia. All patients with PBC should undergo DEXA scan when the diagnosis is first made and every 2 to 4 years thereafter for continuous screening. Counseling your patients regarding healthy nutrition, smoking cessation, and an exercise regimen should also be part of their treatment plan. Treatment for osteoporosis should follow standard guidelines based on T-scores and include the use of calcium, vitamin D supplementation, or the use of bisphosphonates. With respect to hyperlipidemia, current literature does not support any increase risk for cardiovascular disease in patients with PBC. However, for patients with PBC and features of metabolic syndrome, such as hypertension, dyslipidemia, and diabetes, treatment with cholesterol-lowering agents is recommended and not contraindicated.

The most dreaded complication of PBC is progression to end-stage liver disease and the need for liver transplantation. Patients may develop portal hypertension, with appearance of esophageal varices, hepatic encephalopathy, ascites, and are also at risk for hepatocellular carcinoma. These individual complications should be managed according to established guidelines including EGD for variceal screening and ultrasound with or without alpha fetoprotein measurement for HCC screening. Severity of end-stage liver disease should be monitored via the MELD score, and scores of 15 or greater should be referred to expert centers with transplant capabilities.

Conclusion

Primary biliary cholangitis is a progressive autoimmune cholestatic liver disease. Despite rates of liver transplantation for this disease declining since the introduction of UDCA, a significant subset of patients do not respond to therapy and may progress to end-stage liver disease. Recognition of symptoms of PBC in conjunction with effective diagnostic studies, early initiation of treatment with UDCA, and appropriate risk stratification to identify nonresponders in need of adjuvant therapy are essential to prevent the progression to end-stage liver disease and prolong transplant-free survival. Most importantly, evaluation after

1 year of treatment with UDCA is crucial to establish the patient's prognosis and determine the need for changes in the treatment algorithm. PBC patients should be managed holistically with a focus on treatment of disease and its associated coexistent symptoms and offered social support and patient education material to avoid a negative impact on quality of life.

Further Reading

1. Boberg KM, Chapman RW, Hirschfield GM, Lohse AW, Manns MP, Schrumpf E. Overlap syndromes: the international autoimmune hepatitis group (IAIHG) position statement on a controversial issue. J Hepatol. 2011;54(2):374–85.
2. Carey EJ, Ali AH, Lindor KD. Primary biliary cirrhosis. Lancet. 2015;386(10003):1565–75.
3. Corpechot C, Carrat F, Poujol-Robert A, Gaouar F, Wendum D, Chazouillères O, et al. Noninvasive elastography-based assessment of liver fibrosis progression and prognosis in primary biliary cirrhosis. Hepatology. 2012;56(1):198–208.
4. Dufour DR, Lott JA, Nolte FS, Gretch DR, Koff RS, Seeff LB. Diagnosis and monitoring of hepatic injury. II. Recommendations for use of laboratory tests in screening, diagnosis, and monitoring. Clin Chem. 2000;46(12):2050–68.
5. Hirschfield GM, Beuers U, Corpechot C, Invernizzi P, Jones D, Marzioni M, et al. EASL clinical practice guidelines: the diagnosis and management of patients with primary biliary cholangitis. J Hepatol. 2017;67(1):145–72.
6. Kwo PY, Cohen SM, Lim JK. ACG clinical guideline: evaluation of abnormal liver chemistries. Am J Gastroenterol. 2016;112:18.
7. Lammers WJ, van Buuren HR, Hirschfield GM, Janssen HLA, Invernizzi P, Mason AL, et al. Levels of alkaline phosphatase and bilirubin are surrogate end points of outcomes of patients with primary biliary cirrhosis: an international follow-up study. Gastroenterology. 2014;147(6):1338–49. e5.
8. Lindor KD, Gershwin ME, Poupon R, Kaplan M, Bergasa NV, Heathcote EJ. Primary biliary cirrhosis. Hepatology. 2009;50(1):291–308.

Chapter 18
Primary Sclerosing Cholangitis

Shivani Ketan Shah and Marina G. Silveira

Introduction

Primary sclerosing cholangitis (PSC) is a rare, chronic cholestatic liver disease characterized by progressive multifocal strictures of the intra- and extrahepatic bile ducts. Patients are often asymptomatic on presentation, but common symptoms include pruritus, fatigue, and abdominal pain. During the course of the disease, many patients develop recurrent cholangitis, biliary cirrhosis, and end-stage liver disease. No effective medical therapy for PSC is currently available, but ursodeoxycholic acid is commonly used in practice. Ultimately, many patients with PSC may require transplant, after which recurrent disease is a risk. Complications including bacterial cholangitis, fat-soluble vitamin deficiency, metabolic bone diseases, and development of hepatobiliary or colon cancers can occur. In this chapter, we describe a case of primary sclerosing cholangitis in an

S. K. Shah
Yale Traditional Internal Medicine Residency, New Haven, CT, USA
e-mail: shivani.shah@yale.edu

M. G. Silveira (✉)
Yale School of Medicine, New Haven, CT, USA
e-mail: marina.silveira@yale.edu

© Springer Nature Switzerland AG 2019
S. M. Cohen, P. Davitkov (eds.), *Liver Disease*,
https://doi.org/10.1007/978-3-319-98506-0_18

asymptomatic patient. We discuss the differential diagnosis, evaluation, management, and treatment of PSC.

Clinical Case Scenario

A 33-year-old gentleman presented to clinic for further evaluation of a 6-month history of abnormal liver tests. He was asymptomatic, except for fatigue. A complete review of systems was negative for any significant findings. His medical history was significant for a diagnosis of ulcerative colitis since the age of 15, well controlled with mesalamine daily. He had no prior surgeries. He denied the use of any herbal or dietary supplements or over-the-counter medications. He had no history of liver disease or risk factors for chronic liver disease, such as blood transfusions, intravenous drug use, high-risk sexual behavior, or current or past alcohol use. He had not used any tobacco products. His family history was negative for any history of hepatobiliary disorders, autoimmune diseases, or inflammatory bowel disease.

Physical exam revealed a thin gentleman in no distress. There were no stigmata of chronic liver disease. His abdomen was non-distended and nontender. There was no evidence of ascites.

His complete blood count and basic metabolic profile were both unremarkable. His liver blood tests revealed total protein 8.6 g/dL, albumin 4.6 g/dL, alkaline phosphatase 296 U/L, bilirubin 0.4 mg/dL, AST 49 U/L, and ALT 98 U/L. His ultrasound did not reveal any hepatosplenomegaly or focal hepatic lesions. His liver showed normal echogenicity. There was no common bile duct dilation on ultrasound. His gallbladder did not show any evidence of cholelithiasis, sludge, or gallbladder wall thickening. There was no pericholecystic fluid.

Questions

1. What is the differential diagnosis for a patient with chronic cholestasis?
2. What additional tests should be ordered as part of the diagnostic evaluation?
3. What are the diagnostic criteria for PSC?
4. What are the treatment options for PSC?
5. What are the complications of PSC?
6. How do you monitor PSC disease activity?

Discussion

Question 1. What is the differential diagnosis for a patient with chronic cholestasis?

The abnormal liver biochemistries and the history of ulcerative colitis in this patient raise the suspicion for PSC. A cholestatic pattern of liver injury, with a disproportionate elevation of alkaline phosphatase (ALP) level as compared to aminotransferase levels, is the biochemical hallmark of PSC. ALP levels are typically elevated between three and ten times the upper limit of normal, though some patients may have normal ALP levels. Serum alanine and aspartate aminotransferase levels can be between two and three times the upper limit of normal. PSC has the propensity to affect young to middle-aged males and is commonly associated with inflammatory bowel disease, which is present in approximately 70% of patients with PSC. The association between PSC and ulcerative colitis is particularly strong, but patients may also have Crohn's disease and, less frequently, indeterminate colitis. At presentation, most patients are asymptomatic, though progressive symptoms, including fatigue, pruritus, and right upper quadrant pain, can develop as the disease progresses. Less frequently, patients can present with symptoms of complications including bacterial cholangitis, portal hypertension, end-stage liver disease, or hepatobiliary cancers.

A small subgroup of patients with PSC have disease that affects only small intrahepatic bile ducts and thus have normal cholangiograms, also referred to as small duct PSC. Small duct PSC is usually associated with a lower risk of complications and higher survival rates compared to patients with classic PSC. An additional subgroup of patients with PSC may have an overlap syndrome with autoimmune hepatitis (AIH), presenting with concomitant elevations in serum auto-antibodies and a five to ten-fold increase in serum aminotransferase levels. Liver biopsy in these patients typically shows evidence of moderate to severe interface hepatitis. Patients with an overlap syndrome of PSC with AIH may benefit from treatment with steroids, unlike patients with classic PSC.

Primary biliary cholangitis (PBC) is a chronic cholestatic liver disease that predominantly affects middle-aged women. As in PSC, the majority of patients are asymptomatic on presentation, but fatigue or pruritus are common symptoms that develop over the course of the disease. Anti-mitochondrial antibody (AMA) is positive in up to 95% of patients with PBC and is highly specific for the diagnosis in the setting of chronic cholestasis once other causes of intra- and extrahepatic cholestasis are excluded. Liver biopsy is typically reserved for when AMA is absent, if the biochemical profile shows a mixed cholestatic and hepatocellular pattern, or in the setting of other comorbidities such as non-alcoholic steatohepatitis. Liver biopsy may show an intense inflammatory infiltrate centered around the bile ducts, consisting of lymphocytes, plasma cells, macrophages, and polymorphonuclear cells coalesced to a granuloma, and destruction of the interlobular and septal bile ducts, otherwise known as "florid duct lesions." The florid duct lesion is the histological hallmark of PBC but is found in only about 10% of biopsy specimens.

Choledocholithiasis, the presence of stones or debris within the common bile duct, may lead to dilation of the common bile duct. Choledocholithiasis can be detected on ultrasound or magnetic retrograde cholangiopancreatography (MRCP). Treatment is typically with endoscopic retrograde cholangiopancreatography (ERCP). Though choledocholithiasis is typically associated with symptoms including acute abdominal pain, nausea, and vomiting, occasional patients are asymptomatic. Complicated choledocholithiasis can be associated with fevers, hypotension, and mental status changes.

Secondary sclerosing cholangitis can result from ischemia to the biliary tree. Diffuse biliary strictures of intra- or extrahepatic bile ducts can be seen on cholangiograms of patients with ischemic cholangiopathy, usually as a result from recent surgeries including liver transplantation or prolonged intensive care unit stays. IgG4-associated cholangitis is a systemic condition difficult to distinguish from PSC by biochemical testing or imaging studies alone. It is characterized by markedly elevated levels of serum IgG4 and lymphoplasmacytic infiltrates of the affected organs, such as bile ducts and pancreas, which are IgG4 positive on special staining studies. It is important to distinguish IgG4-associated cholangitis from PSC, as it often responds to therapy with steroids, unlike PSC. Table 18.1 includes and summarizes the differential diagnosis of secondary sclerosing cholangitis.

Table 18.1 Etiologies of secondary sclerosing cholangitis

Secondary sclerosing cholangitis
Choledocholithiasis
Cholangiocarcinoma
IgG4-associated cholangitis
Ischemic cholangitis
Histiocytosis X
Portal hypertensive biliopathy
Recurrent pancreatitis
Surgical biliary trauma
Diffuse intrahepatic metastasis
AIDS cholangiopathy

Malignancy including cholangiocarcinoma (CCA) can also mimic PSC.

Question 2. What additional tests should be ordered as part of the diagnostic evaluation?

This young, asymptomatic male shows the biochemical signs of cholestasis. To further evaluate the etiology of cholestasis, serologies and imaging should be performed.

In order to exclude immune-mediated liver diseases, such as PBC, and AIH, serological tests aiming at detecting AMA, antinuclear antibodies (ANA), smooth muscle antibodies (SMA), and immunoglobulin levels should be performed. Ceruloplasmin, ferritin, and alpha-1-antitrypsin levels should be determined to exclude hereditary etiologies of liver disease such as Wilson's disease, hereditary hemochromatosis, and alpha-1-antitrypsin deficiency. Chronic viral hepatitis should be excluded. To assess for secondary sclerosing cholangitis, IgG4 levels and CA19-9 should be obtained to evaluate for IgG4-associated cholangitis and CCA, respectively.

PSC has no diagnostic serum autoantibody tests. Multiple autoantibodies can be detected in patients with PSC, which are typically not disease specific. The prevalence of antibodies in PSC widely varies. Atypical perinuclear antineutrophil cytoplasmic antibodies (ANCA) are positive in 25–95% of patients but lack in diagnostic specificity. Other autoantibodies include ANA, present in 7–77% of patients, and SMA, described in 13–20% of patients, which are usually in lower titers than those observed in AIH. In contrast, a positive AMA is seldom seen in patients with PSC.

Abdominal imaging should be done at the onset of abnormal liver biochemistries to exclude biliary obstruction and secondary sclerosing cholangitis and to assess for signs of advanced fibrosis or portal hypertension. Abdominal ultrasound is helpful in excluding biliary stones and obvious masses. Cross-sectional imaging with contrasted CT or MRI is used for the diagnosis and staging of suspected cholangiocarcinoma, but the sensitivity is low. MRCP is the standard investigation for the diagnosis of PSC. As seen in Fig. 18.1, a beading appearance caused by short multifocal strictures of the intrahepatic or extrahepatic bile ducts, or both, is characteristic. MRCP has been shown to have a high sensitivity and very high specificity for the diagnosis of PSC. The disadvantage to MRCP is that biopsies or interventions of the strictures cannot be performed.

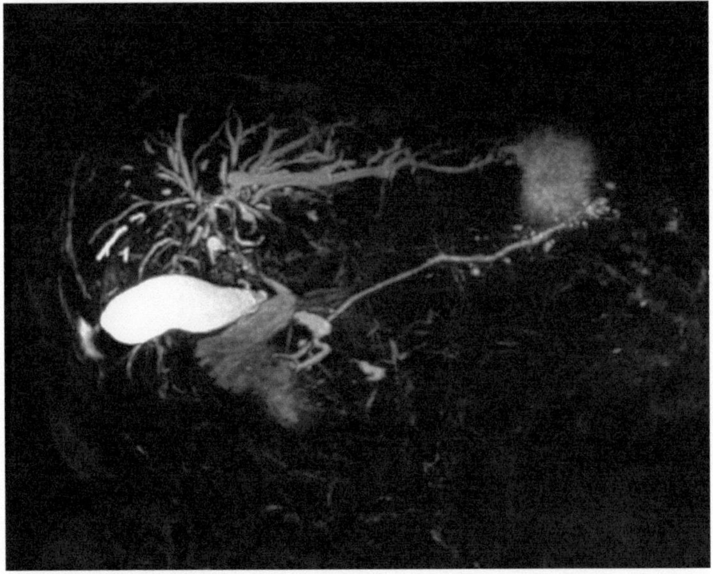

Fig. 18.1 MRCP showing multifocal stricturing of intrahepatic ducts, characteristic of PSC

ERCP, once the standard investigation for the diagnosis of PSC, is now reserved for therapeutic intervention or assessment of bile duct strictures. Clinical scenarios in which ERCP should be considered include a dominant stricture on MRCP, high suspicion of choledocholithiasis or cholangitis, or, infrequently, if the patient is unable to tolerate MRCP. If stones are found, a sphincterotomy may be performed to help alleviate the obstruction and drain the bile duct. If strictures are found, balloon dilation may be performed and/or stents may be placed. Brush cytology and biopsies of the bile duct can be taken when there is suspicion of cholangiocarcinoma. ERCP is associated with risks of complications, including those associated with sedation, as well as procedure-related risks, such as pancreatitis, infections, and bowel perforation.

If the cholangiogram is normal but small-duct PSC is suspected or if the aminotransferase levels are greater than five times the upper limit of normal and overlap with AIH is suspected, a liver biopsy may be indicated. The classical histological finding of PSC is concentric, periductal "onion-skin" fibrosis (shown in Fig. 18.2),

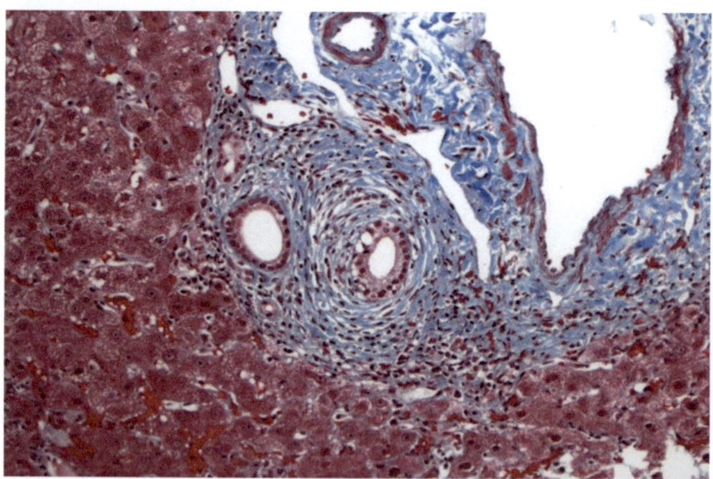

Fig. 18.2 Periductal "onion-skin" fibrosis (Magnification, ×200; Trichrome stain). (Image courtesy of Dhanpat Jain, MD. Yale School of Medicine, Yale University, New Haven, CT)

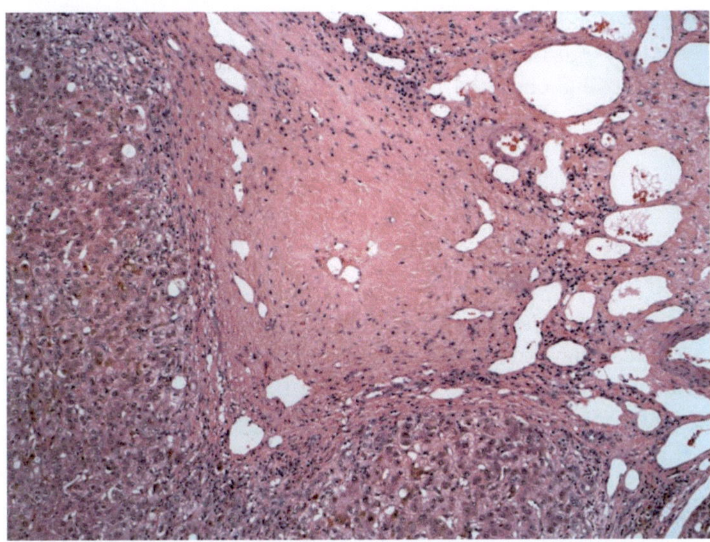

Fig. 18.3 Completely obliterated bile duct with periductal fibrosis, no visible epithelium. (Magnification ×200; Tomb-stone lesion; H&E stain). (Image courtesy of Dhanpat Jain, MD. Yale School of Medicine, Yale University, New Haven, CT)

but this is often not found in biopsy specimens, particularly in early-stage disease. Bile duct obliteration (shown in Fig. 18.3) may also be present on biopsy but is also nonspecific. Approximately 98% of patients with PSC may have no typical histological findings on liver biopsy, limiting the diagnostic utility of a liver biopsy.

Question 3. What are the diagnostic criteria for PSC?

A diagnosis of PSC is typically established based on the key aspects of chronic cholestasis (persistent for more than 6 months) in conjunction with bile duct changes such as strictures and dilatations on cholangiography (mainly detected by MRCP but infrequently requiring ERCP). Secondary causes of sclerosing cholangitis, as detailed in Table 18.1, must be excluded.

Clinical Case: Continued

Our patient underwent additional lab testing. His ANA, SMA AMA, ceruloplasmin, alpha-1-antitrypsin, ferritin, hepatitis serologies, IgG levels, IgG4 levels, and CA 19-9 tests were all negative or within normal limits.

Our patient also underwent an MRCP that showed diffuse multifocal strictures of the intrahepatic and extrahepatic bile ducts (including the common bile duct). In the setting of cholestasis in the context of chronic ulcerative colitis, normal immunoglobulins, negative autoimmune, and tumor markers, a diagnosis of PSC was established.

Question 4. What are the treatment options for PSC?

There currently is no effective medical therapy for PSC.

Ursodeoxycholic acid (UDCA) is frequently used in patients with PSC, often around doses of 20 mg/kg/day. However, there is no clear evidence that UDCA slows the progression to cirrhosis, liver transplant, and death, despite improvement of liver biochemistries. High doses of UDCA (28–30 mg/kg) have been associated with substantially more adverse outcomes, such as the need for transplantation and the development of varices, as well an increased risk of colorectal neoplasia in the context of ulcerative colitis, despite improvement of ALP levels, and therefore should not be used.

Many other treatments including immunosuppressant agents have been evaluated but have not been shown to have any proven clinical benefit in PSC.

Selected patients with dominant strictures, which is a stenosis that is <1.5 mm in the common bile duct or <1.0 mm in the hepatic duct, may benefit from endoscopic intervention. ERCP may relieve the complications of pruritus and cholangitis, allow diagnosis of cholangiocarcinoma, and may lead to improved survival. Techniques employed for endoscopic therapy are not well standardized and include dilatation, stenting, and combinations of these methods. Stent placement may be associated with higher treatment-related complications, such as cholangitis. Prophylactic antibiotic therapy is recommended for patients undergoing ERCP.

In patients with decompensated cirrhosis, liver transplantation (LT) is recommended for eligible patients. PSC is the fourth most common diagnosis for LT in the United States. LT should also be considered in patients with intractable pruritus and recurrent cholangitis. The Model for End-Stage Liver Disease (MELD) score is a general LT allocation instrument that predicts 3-month mortality in end-stage liver disease; ACG guidelines suggest that a MELD of greater than 14 warrants a referral to LT. Recurrent episodes of cholangitis (>2 episodes of bacteremia or >1 episode of sepsis), CCA <3 cm in diameter and no evidence of metastasis currently undergoing treatment through an IRB-approved clinical trial, or intractable pruritus may allow for a patient to receive MELD exception points with the United Network for Organ Sharing Regional Review Board. LT offers 90% 1-year survival rates and 70–85% 5-year survival rates in PSC. PSC recurrence after LT is evident in approximately 8–27% of patients.

Question 5. What are the complications of PSC?

PSC is associated with several complications, ranging from systemic symptoms of fatigue and pruritus, increased risk of hepatobiliary, and colorectal malignancy to end-stage liver disease and its complications. Table 18.2 summarizes the common complications of PSC as well as recommended management.

Table 18.2 Complications associated with PSC and the evaluation and management of the complications by the American Association for the Study of Liver Diseases (AASLD) and the American College of Gastroenterology (ACG)

Complication	AASLD[a]	ACG
Dominant stricture	1. ERCP for evaluation (1B) 2. Treatment of dominant strictures via dilatation or stenting (1B) 3. Brush cytology and/or biopsy of dominant strictures to screen for malignancy (1B)	1. ERCP is recommended for PSC with dominant stricture (strong recommendation, low quality of evidence) 2. Dominant strictures should have ERCP with cytology, biopsies, and FISH to screen for malignancy (strong recommendation, low quality of evidence)
Cholangitis	1. Prophylactic antibiotics if the patient has recurrent cholangitis (1B) 2. Liver transplant evaluation for refractory bacterial cholangitis (1B)	1. Antibiotic prophylaxis to prevent post-ERCP cholangitis (conditional recommendation, low quality of evidence)
Bone mineral disease	1. Bone mineral density screening at time of diagnosis and 2–3-year intervals (1B)	1. Bone mineral density screening at time of diagnosis and at 2–4-year intervals (conditional recommendation, moderate quality of evidence)

Table 18.2 (continued)

Complication	AASLD[a]	ACG
Cholangiocarcinoma (CCA)	1. Screening for CCA should be performed if patients have deterioration in constitutional performance or worsening biochemical-related parameters (1B) 2. If the patient has CCA and no evidence of cirrhosis, attempt surgical resection (2B) 3. If early CCA is not amenable to surgical resection, consider evaluating patient for liver transplant (1B)	1. Consider screening for CCA with regular imaging (ultrasound or MR) plus CA 19-9 every 6–12 months (conditional recommendation, very low quality of evidence)
Gallbladder malignancy	1. Perform annual ultrasound to detect mass lesions in the gallbladder (1C) 2. If a gallbladder mass is present, cholecystectomy should be performed, regardless of size (1C)	1. Cholecystectomy is recommended for patients with gallbladder polyps >8 mm (conditional recommendation, very low quality of evidence)

(continued)

Table 18.2 (continued)

Complication	AASLD[a]	ACG
Colorectal Cancer	1. If the patient has PSC and no evidence of inflammatory bowel disease at time of diagnosis, perform full colonoscopy with biopsies (1A) 2. If the patient has inflammatory bowel disease and PSC, perform surveillance colonoscopies at 1–2 year intervals (1B) 3. Do not use UDCA as chemoprevention for colorectal cancer (1B)	1. If the patient has PSC and no evidence of inflammatory bowel disease, perform a full colonoscopy with biopsies (conditional recommendation, moderate quality of evidence) 2. Annual colon surveillance with chromoendoscopy should be performed in patients with primary sclerosing cholangitis and inflammatory bowel disease at the time of diagnosis (conditional recommendations, moderate quality of evidence)
Cirrhosis/advanced liver disease	1. Patients with advanced liver disease should be considered for liver transplant as a successful treatment modality (1A)	1. Liver transplant is recommended over medical therapy or surgical drainage in PSC patients with decompensated cirrhosis (strong recommendation, moderate quality of evidence) 2. Refer for liver transplant when MELD (Model for End-Stage Liver Disease) is >14

[a]AASLD guidelines are based on Grading of Recommendations, Assessment, Development and Evaluations (GRADE) Working Group, with *1* indicating a strong recommendation, *2* indicating a weak recommendation, *A* indicating high quality of evidence for the recommendation, *B* indicating moderate quality of evidence, and *C* indicating low quality of evidence

Patients with PSC are often asymptomatic on presentation, but progressive symptoms, such as fatigue and pruritus, develop during the course of the disease. No therapy is available for fatigue. In patients with pruritus, first-line medical therapy for pruritus is the bile acid sequestrant cholestyramine. Second-line therapies include rifampin, naltrexone, and sertraline. In patients with pruritus and a dominant stricture, endoscopic intervention should be considered.

A dominant stricture is a stenosis that is <1.5 mm in the common bile duct or <1.0 mm in the hepatic duct that can occur in PSC and is associated with an increased risk of cholangiocarcinoma. A dominant stricture can be associated with cholangitis and may be treated by ERCP.

Bone mineral disease is a common complication of patients with chronic cholestasis, including patients with PSC. Fat-soluble vitamin deficiencies may occur in patients with PSC, particularly in the late stages of the disease.

PSC is also associated with an increased risk of hepatobiliary malignancies, particularly CCA and gallbladder cancer. An approximate 20% lifetime risk of CCA is estimated in PSC. CA19-9 measurements are traditionally used for screening but lack sensitivity and specificity for diagnosis, although evidence suggests utility in combination with imaging modalities. MRCP, combined with contrast-enhanced MRI of the liver, or ERCP with brush cytology and/or biopsies can be used for diagnosis, though the definitive diagnosis of CCA can be challenging. There is also an increased risk of gallbladder cancer; though the true risk is unknown, one study suggested that 40–60% of gallbladder masses in patients with PSC are malignant.

Patients with IBD and PSC are also at an increased risk of colorectal cancer, with an estimated incidence of approximately 30% at 20 years after diagnosis of PSC.

Question 6. How do you monitor PSC disease activity?

Patients with PSC should be monitored closely after initial diagnosis. The natural history of PSC, though highly variable, is progressive, evolving through biliary fibrosis to liver cirrhosis and end-stage liver disease or CCA in the vast majority of patients. Though patients are often asymptomatic at the time of diagnosis, patients often develop symptoms over time. Liver biochemistries, including ALP and bilirubin, naturally fluctuate over time, with transient elevations precipitated by cholangitis, biliary calculi, or dominant strictures. Routine liver biochemistries should be performed every 3–6 months. Normalization of ALP levels, independent of the use of UDCA, is associated with a better prognosis, including decreased risk of neoplasia, liver transplant, or death. Patients should be monitored for the complications highlighted in Table 18.2.

Several attempts have been made to develop a PSC-specific risk stratification or prognostic model. The most widely used model is the revised Mayo risk score, which is based on age, bilirubin, albumin, AST, and variceal bleeding. Once patients develop cirrhosis, general cirrhosis scores such as the Child-Pugh score may be used for staging and prognostication but are less useful than the revised Mayo risk score in patients with less advanced disease. The 7-year survival rates in PSC cirrhosis patients with Child-Pugh scores of A, B, and C are approximately 90%, 70%, and 25%, respectively.

The enhanced liver fibrosis (ELF) score testing and elastography are noninvasive tests of liver fibrosis used for stratification and prognostication in PSC. The ELF test is a serum study based on components of fibrogenesis and matrix remodeling. There is evidence showing that ELF can independently predict clinical outcomes of liver transplant or death in patients with PSC. Transient elastography (TE) is an ultrasound-based modality that examines liver stiffness measurements (LSM), thus providing a surrogate for estimating degree of fibrosis within the liver parenchyma. Studies on liver TE suggest strong correlations with degree of fibrosis on histology and LSM, particularly in higher degrees of fibrosis in patients with PSC. An association between clinical outcome and both baseline LSM and changes in LSM has been demonstrated for TE and may be useful for monitoring of patients with PSC.

PSC is a progressive disease, ultimately leading to the development of portal hypertension and cirrhosis. Complications of portal hypertension include thrombocytopenia, ascites, encephalopathy, and gastroesophageal varices and generally are not unique to PSC. Patients with PSC who have an ileal stoma after colectomy sustain an increased rate of bleeding from peristomal varices. Imaging and endoscopic modalities may be useful in monitoring for portal hypertension and cirrhosis. Changes in hepatic morphology as detected by MRI, particularly atrophy, can be associated with liver transplant and all-cause mortality.

Conclusion

PSC is a chronic, cholestatic liver disease involving the intra- and extrahepatic bile ducts. A diagnosis is established based on biochemical studies in conjunction with imaging studies. There are no current effective treatment options for PSC, but UDCA in low to moderate doses is frequently used. Disease activity may be monitored through serum biochemistries, ELF score, and liver elastography, and prognostication can be performed with the revised Mayo risk score. Patients may experience complications such as pruritus, bone mineral disease, recurrent cholangitis, dominant strictures, hepatobiliary malignancies, and may ultimately require LT, which is curative, but disease recurrence is a concern.

Further Reading

1. Boonstra K, Weersma RK, van Erpecum KJ, Rauws EA, Spanier BW, Poen AC, et al. Population-based epidemiology, malignancy risk, and outcome of primary sclerosing cholangitis. Hepatology. 2013;58(6):2045–55.
2. Chapman R, Fevery J, Kalloo A, Nagorney DM, Boberg KM, Shneider B, et al. Diagnosis and management of primary sclerosing cholangitis. Hepatology. 2010;51(2):660–78.
3. Dave M, Elmunzer BJ, Dwamena BA, Higgins PD. Primary sclerosing cholangitis: meta-analysis of diagnostic performance of MR cholangio-pancreatography. Radiology. 2010;256(2):387–96.
4. Karlsen TH, Folseraas T, Thorburn D, Vesterhus M. Primary sclerosing cholangitis – a comprehensive review. J Hepatol. 2017;67(6):1298–323.
5. Lindor KD, Kowdley KV, Harrison ME. American College of G. ACG clinical guideline: primary sclerosing cholangitis. Am J Gastroenterol. 2015;110(5):646–59; quiz 60.
6. Singh S, Talwalkar JA. Primary sclerosing cholangitis: diagnosis, prognosis, and management. Clin Gastroenterol Hepatol. 2013;11(8):898–907.
7. Visseren T, Darwish MS. Recurrence of primary sclerosing cholangitis, primary biliary cholangitis and auto-immune hepatitis after liver transplantation. Best Pract Res Clin Gastroenterol. 2017;31(2):187–98.

Chapter 19
General Overview of the Liver Transplant Patient

Anjana Pillai and Thomas Couri

Introduction

Liver transplantation (LT) is the only cure for end-stage liver disease. Almost 6000 liver transplants were performed in 2013, and more than 15,000 patients are on the liver transplant waiting list in the United States. Patient outcomes continue to improve with the majority of patients living more than 10 years after LT. With this increased life expectancy, attention to the long-term care of liver transplant recipients is paramount. In this chapter, we discuss the common medical conditions, the immunosuppression and antimicrobial prophylaxis regimens, and the approach to abnormal liver chemistry tests in the LT recipient.

A. Pillai (✉)
Division of Gastroenterology, Hepatology, and Nutrition,
University of Chicago Medical Center, Chicago, IL, USA
e-mail: apillai1@medicine.bsd.uchicago.edu

T. Couri
Department of Internal Medicine, University of Chicago Medical
Center, Chicago, IL, USA

© Springer Nature Switzerland AG 2019
S. M. Cohen, P. Davitkov (eds.), *Liver Disease*,
https://doi.org/10.1007/978-3-319-98506-0_19

Clinical Case Scenario

A 55-year-old man with a history of alcohol-related cirrhosis and subsequent orthotopic liver transplant (LT) presents to his primary care provider (PCP) for a routine visit 3 months after his LT. He had an unremarkable postoperative course. He denies any alcohol use in over a year and denies any cravings. He had a colonoscopy at age 51 that was normal. He has no other pertinent medical history. He is currently taking tacrolimus, low-dose prednisone, trimethoprim-sulfamethoxazole, and valganciclovir. He has gained 15 pounds since his last visit 4 months ago, and his body mass index (BMI) is 31.0 kg/m². His vital signs are remarkable for a blood pressure of 155/95. His physical exam is otherwise unremarkable except for a well-healed surgical scar on his abdomen.

Questions

1. What medical problems are LT recipients at risk for?
2. What are common immunosuppression medications for post-LT patients?
3. What antimicrobial prophylaxis is appropriate for post-LT patients?
4. What is the differential diagnosis for and approach to abnormal liver chemistry tests in the LT patient?

Discussion

Question 1. What medical problems are LT recipients at risk for?

LT recipients are expected to have continued improvements in survival (>90% at 1 year and >75% at 5 years) due to improvements in both surgical techniques and immunosuppression regimens. This increased survival benefit is countered by several expected posttransplant complications largely caused by immunosuppressants (Table 19.1). Physicians should be aware of the higher incidence of the metabolic syndrome and its associated

Table 19.1 Diseases that commonly affect the LT patient

Disease	Screening interval	Diagnosis	Treatment
Obesity	Every visit	BMI >30.0 kg/m^2	[a]Dietary modifications, exercise, minimize or discontinue offending medications, bariatric surgery
Dyslipidemia	Annual lipid panel	Elevated LDL or triglycerides or decreased HDL	Dietary modifications, exercise, weight loss, tobacco cessation, statin therapy if indicated
Diabetes mellitus	Every 3 months for 1 year, then annually, with hemoglobin A1c measurement or FBG	Hemoglobin A1c of >6.4% or FBG of >125 mg/dL on two occasions	Dietary modifications, exercise, weight loss, minimize or discontinue offending medications, insulin or oral DM agents
Hypertension	Every visit	Blood pressure >130/80	Dietary modifications, <1500 mg salt per day, exercise, weight loss, amlodipine then ACEI/ARB or beta-blocker if tolerated

(continued)

                                                                    A. Pillai and T. Couri

Table 19.1 (continued)

Disease	Screening interval	Diagnosis	Treatment
Nonalcoholic fatty liver disease	Unclear	Steatosis on imaging, +/− elevated transaminases if other causes excluded; biopsy gold standard	Dietary modifications including addition of olive oil and coffee, exercise, weight loss[a]
Cardiovascular disease	Unclear	Clinical diagnosis (based upon imaging, stress testing, or clinical event)	Dietary modifications, exercise, weight loss, tobacco cessation, statin therapy, aspirin for primary prevention if indicated
Chronic kidney disease	Annual GFR calculation and urine protein to creatinine ratio	GFR <60 mL/min/1.73 m^2 for 3 or more months	Discontinue or minimize offending medications, optimize DM and hypertension treatment

BMI body mass index, *FBG* fasting blood glucose, *DM* diabetes mellitus, *mg* milligrams, *ACEI* angiotensin-converting enzyme inhibitor, *ARB* angiotensin receptor blocker, *GFR* glomerular filtration rate
[a]The Mediterranean diet is currently the most accepted dietary recommendation

conditions, chronic kidney disease, and malignancy in posttransplant patients.

The incidence of the metabolic syndrome—obesity, dyslipidemia, insulin resistance, hyperglycemia, and hypertension—increases and is a significant risk factor for morbidity and mortality after LT. Approximately one-third of patients who were not obese pretransplant become obese posttransplant.

Possible etiologies of posttransplant obesity include medication side effects (particularly immunosuppression medications), increased incidence of diabetes, and increased nutritional intake. The patient in this clinical scenario has become obese since his transplant. He should be screened for other components of the metabolic syndrome and be advised on dietary modifications and to exercise at least 150 minutes per week. Steroids should be weaned or discontinued when possible. Orlistat, a weight loss medication, has not been shown to be effective in improving BMI and may alter immunosuppression medication levels. Bariatric surgery has been shown to be effective in LT patients.

Dyslipidemia affects 45–69% of LT patients, and its incidence increases posttransplant. Many immunosuppression agents used in LT patients cause elevated cholesterol and triglyceride levels, particularly steroids, sirolimus and everolimus. All LT patients should be screened annually with a lipid panel. Dietary modifications such as adherence to the Mediterranean diet or a diet low in saturated fats and cholesterol should be advised for patients with dyslipidemia. Hepatologists have recommended statin pharmacotherapy if the low-density lipoprotein (LDL) level is greater than 130 mg/dL. However, newer guidelines from the American College of Cardiology and the American Heart Association recommend statin therapy if atherosclerotic cardiovascular disease (ASCVD) is present, if LDL is greater or equal to 190 mg/dL, if a patient has diabetes and is between 40 and 75 years old, or if the 10-year ASCVD risk as assessed by the Pooled Cohort Equations is greater or equal to 7.5% in patients 40–75 years old. Pravastatin, which has been shown to be safe and well tolerated in LT patients, has been the pharmacotherapy studied most and does not depend on the cytochrome p450 CYP3A4 pathway for metabolism. Other statins which use this pathway have been shown to increase levels of calcineurin inhibitors (tacrolimus and cyclosporine), although without clinical side effects.

Diabetes mellitus (DM) prevalence before LT is estimated at 1–25%, and 20–37% of patients develop new-onset DM after LT. New-onset DM after LT develops quickly for most patients, with 80% of patients developing DM within 1 month posttransplant. Immunosuppression agents, specifically steroids and calcineurin inhibitors, cause increased insulin resistance and diabetes. Multiple studies have documented the adverse effects of DM on LT patients, including increased rates of hepatic artery thrombosis, graft fibrosis, and mortality. LT patients should be screened every 3 months for DM with either a fasting blood glucose or hemoglobin A1c and then annually thereafter. Treatment is similar to all patients with DM and includes a diet low in saturated fats and cholesterol, regular physical activity, and weight loss. Steroids should be discontinued if possible or, if unable, weaned to the lowest dose tolerated. DM medications have not been studied specifically in LT patients; however, some experts have proposed treating normal or underweight patients with insulin and overweight patients with oral DM medications. Sulfonylureas and rosiglitazone are safe in LT patients; however, metformin should be avoided in patients with kidney disease. Cyclosporine, rather than tacrolimus, can be considered as first-line immunosuppression due to the increased incidence of new-onset DM with tacrolimus as compared to cyclosporine in patients at high risk for developing DM. Assessments of glycemic control should be made every 3 months after diagnosis, yearly ophthalmologic and podiatry care should be scheduled, and annual microalbuminuria screening should be done in all DM patients.

Hypertension is rare prior to LT but very common afterwards. As many as 70% of LT recipients develop hypertension, using the prior standard definition of a blood pressure of greater or equal to 140/90. However, we favor using newer guidelines that define hypertension as blood pressure >130/80. Hypertension post-LT develops due to increased systemic vasoconstriction and renal vasoconstriction, the latter of which is increased by calcineurin inhibitors. Blood pressure should be checked at every clinic visit for LT patients, and first-line therapy is dihydropyridine calcium channel blockers such as amlodipine. Nifedipine and non-dihydropyridine calcium channel blockers such as diltiazem should be avoided because they can cause elevated serum levels of calcineurin inhibitors. Suggested second-line therapies include angiotensin-converting enzyme (ACE) inhibitors, angiotensin receptor blockers (ARBs), or beta-blockers. Diuretics are generally not recommended due to the risk of electrolyte derangements. The goal blood pressure target is less than 120/80.

LT patients are at risk for other diseases associated with the metabolic syndrome, including nonalcoholic fatty liver disease (NAFLD) and cardiovascular disease. New-onset NAFLD and nonalcoholic steatohepatitis (NASH) occur in approximately 20% and 10% of LT patients, respectively. For patients who were transplanted due to NASH or cryptogenic cirrhosis, almost 100% of patients will develop steatosis 5 years after LT. Elevated liver transaminases and steatosis on imaging, along with ruling out other causes of chronic liver disease, are the cornerstones of diagnosis, although liver biopsy remains the gold standard. Weight loss, 150 minutes of physical activity per week, Mediterranean diet, olive oil, and at least 2–4 cups of coffee per day have been associated with improvements in NAFLD. The Mediterranean diet consists of liberal amounts of vegetables and non-refined cereals, with modest amounts of dairy, fish, and poultry. Olive oil serves as the principal source of fat, and animal fats are avoided.

Cardiovascular disease is the leading cause of late-term mortality in LT patients. There is an overall 13.6% risk and a 64% increased risk for LT patients compared to non-LT patients of a cardiovascular event, such as acute coronary syndrome or arrhythmia. Hypertension, DM, smoking, sedentary lifestyle, obesity, male gender, advanced age, renal failure, and dyslipidemia are risk factors for cardiovascular disease in LT patients.

Optimization of these diseases and risk factors is the mainstay of treatment. Low-dose aspirin is recommended for primary prevention of cardiovascular disease for patients aged 50–59 with a 10-year ASCVD risk of 10% or greater according to the US Preventive Services Task Force.

Chronic kidney disease (CKD) is a common diagnosis in LT patients and is associated with an increased risk of death. Posttransplant glomerular filtration rate (GFR) decreases to 60% of pretransplant GFR by 6 weeks post-LT. The incidence of chronic renal failure is about 10% at 1 year and 25% at 10 years for LT patients. The etiologies of CKD in LT patients are often the increased rates of hypertension and DM and the use of calcineurin inhibitors. Patients should be assessed with regular measurements of the GFR and annual urinary albumin to creatinine ratios. The treatment of CKD in this population involves aggressive control of the comorbid conditions that worsen CKD—hypertension and DM—and either reducing or switching calcineurin inhibitor immunosuppression for less nephrotoxic agents, such as mycophenolate mofetil or sirolimus.

Malignancy occurs almost 12 times more in LT patients compared to the general population. The incidence of new malignancies after LT is as high as 26%, with a cumulative risk of 11–20% 10 years after LT, and death from malignancy is the second leading cause of late-term death in LT patients. Advancing age, tobacco use, alcohol use, and infection with oncogenic viruses such as hepatitis C virus (HCV) increase the risk of malignancy post-LT. Immunosuppression with tacrolimus increases the risk of solid organ internal cancers, while cyclosporine and azathioprine increase the incidence of skin cancers.

The most common solid organ malignancy after LT is posttransplant lymphoproliferative disorder (PTLD), which occurs in 2–4% of patients. Epstein-Barr virus (EBV) infection of B lymphocytes is thought to trigger cell proliferation and cause PTLD. The highest incidence of PTLD occurs within 18 months of liver transplant, with a cumulative incidence of 5.4%

approximately 20 years after transplant. PTLD more commonly develops earlier in pediatric patients as compared to adults. Patient presentation varies widely but can include fevers, cytopenias, lymphadenopathy, gastrointestinal or pulmonary symptoms, or central nervous system abnormalities. Tissue biopsy is required for diagnosis. Forty five to seventy percent of patients respond to immunosuppression reduction, and those who do not respond require chemotherapy, antibody therapy, radiation, or surgery.

Both non-melanoma cutaneous malignancies and melanoma are increased in LT patients. Squamous cell carcinoma has an incidence 35.7 times higher, and melanoma incidence is 2.8 times higher than in the general population. It is thought that cumulative immunosuppression treatment puts LT patients at greater risk for cutaneous cancers, as well as sun exposure and advancing age. Because of this increased risk, LT patients should receive annual skin exams by a dermatologist, in addition to limiting direct sun exposure, wearing clothes and items that shield patients from the sun, and using sunscreen with a minimum sun protection factor (SPF) of 15.

The primary disease for which the patient was transplanted plays a role in assessing the patient's risk for malignancy. Patients transplanted for alcohol-related cirrhosis have a greater risk for head and neck and esophageal malignancies. No strict guidelines exist; however, some experts recommend yearly ear, nose, and throat (ENT) evaluation for these patients. Patients transplanted for primary sclerosing cholangitis (PSC), which is often associated with ulcerative colitis, are at increased risk for colorectal cancers and should undergo annual screening colonoscopies; colonoscopies every 5 years can be considered generally for other LT patients. Annual anogenital exams for women and high-risk men and Pap smears for female patients are encouraged due to the increased risks of anogenital cancers in LT patients, secondary to HPV infection in the setting of immunosuppression. Other malignancy screening guidelines

Table 19.2 Unique cancer screening recommendations in OLT patients

Malignancy	Screening recommendation
Skin cancer	Annual skin exam by dermatologist
Head and neck cancer	Consider annual ENT evaluation
Colorectal cancer	Consider colonoscopy every 5 years; annually in patients with PSC
Anal cancer	Annual anal exam in women and high-risk men
Cervical cancer	Annual Pap smear
Breast cancer	Annual screening mammogram for all women starting at age 40; men based on family history
Prostate cancer	Individualized decision for screening with prostate-specific antigen for all men age 55–69

recommended for the general population apply to LT patients. Table 19.2 summarizes the specialized recommendations on cancer screening for the LT patient.

Question 2. What are common immunosuppression medications for post-LT patients?

Immunosuppression regimens post-LT vary by institution and provider preference but can be divided into five different categories: corticosteroids, antibody therapy, calcineurin inhibitors (CNIs), mammalian target of rapamycin inhibitors (MTOR-Is), and purine synthesis inhibitors. Corticosteroids are used perioperatively and are often weaned off by 3 months in the majority of patients due their burdensome side effect profile. About 25% of liver transplant centers use antibody therapy—IL-2 receptor antibody antagonists such as daclizumab or basiliximab or antithymocyte globulin—for induction immunosuppression. Improvements in acute cellular rejection and patient survival rates are heavily attributed to the CNIs, cyclosporine and tacrolimus, which remain the cornerstone of immunosuppression for LT patients. Patients taking tacrolimus have been shown to have less rejection compared to those taking cyclosporine, although there are no differences in graft and patient survival between the CNIs (17). The MTOR-Is, sirolimus and everolimus, are believed to increase immune tolerance, have anti-neoplastic properties, and increase renal protection compared to CNIs, although studies have been mixed on these topics. Mycophenolate mofetil and azathioprine are agents in the purine synthesis inhibitor class.

Maintenance or long-term immunosuppression typically involves a CNI agent or MTOR-I, with the possible addition of a purine synthesis inhibitor. An exception is patients who were transplanted for autoimmune hepatitis, who will often remain on steroids for longer periods of time compared to other LT recipients. About 20–30% of patients will achieve full withdrawal of immunosuppression without adverse effects. The hepatologist's decision to wean immunosuppression has to be carefully executed with frequent monitoring of laboratory parameters and depends on a host of factors, including the etiology of primary liver disease, the time from transplant, the age of the patient, and the history of previous rejection episodes.

There are multiple side effects associated with the various immunosuppressant agents. Table 19.3 lists some of the more common side effects seen with these medications. Primary care providers should be aware of these potential adverse effects. In addition, there can be significant drug-drug interactions seen with these agents, especially with the calcineurin inhibitors. Table 19.4 lists some of the more common medications that can result in increased or decreased calcineurin inhibitor levels. Again, primary care providers must be aware of potential interactions of other medications with calcineurin inhibitors.

Table 19.3 Common side effects seen with antirejection immunosuppressants

Immunosuppression side effects			
Calcineurin inhibitors	Azathioprine	Mycophenolate	Sirolimus
Nephrotoxicity	Leukopenia	Leukopenia	Hyperlipidemia
Hepatotoxicity	Anemia	Anemia	Hypertension
Hypertension	Thrombocytopenia	Thrombocytopenia	Leukopenia
Diabetes	Hepatotoxicity	Hepatotoxicity	Anemia
Hyperlipidemia	Cholestasis	Diarrhea	Thrombocytopenia
Neurotoxicity	Pancreatitis	Abdominal pain	Proteinuria
Malignancy	Abdominal pain	Nausea	Interstitial pneumonitis
	Malignancy	Bloating	Delayed wound healing
		Vomiting	Malignancy
		Malignancy	Hepatic artery thrombosis

Table 19.4 Medications that can increase or decrease calcineurin inhibitor levels

Medications that can result in *increased* calcineurin inhibitor levels	Medications that can result in *decreased* calcineurin inhibitor levels
Calcium channel blockers	Antituberculosis agents
Verapamil	Rifampin
Diltiazem	Rifabutin
Amlodipine	Isoniazid
Nicardipine	Anticonvulsants
Antifungal agents	Barbiturates
Ketoconazole	Phenytoin
Fluconazole	Carbamazepine
Itraconazole	St. John's wort
Clotrimazole	Antibiotics
Sirolimus	Nafcillin
Glucocorticoids	Imipenem
Antibiotics	Cephalosporins
Erythromycin	Terbinafine
Clarithromycin	Ciprofloxacin
Azithromycin	Ticlopidine
Protease inhibitors	Octreotide
Saquinavir	
Indinavir	
Nelfinavir	
Ritonavir	
Grapefruit and grapefruit juice	

Question 3. What antimicrobial prophylaxis is appropriate for post-LT patients?

Antimicrobials are universally used for prophylaxis in the post-LT setting. Trimethoprim-sulfamethoxazole is used for 4 to 12 months post-LT to prevent *Pneumocystis jirovecii* infection. More than 70% of transplant centers use valganciclovir to prevent cytomegalovirus (CMV) infection or reactivation. Transplant centers vary on the length of CMV prophylaxis treatment, with some experts recommending 3–6 months of valganciclovir for high-risk patients (donor positive and recipient negative (D+/R-)) and 3 months for intermediate-risk patients (D+/R+). Patients who are seronegative for varicella zoster virus (VZV) should receive VZV immunization pretransplant and should receive antiviral prophylaxis if exposed posttransplant and without seroconversion. Acyclovir for herpes simplex virus (HSV) prophylaxis has also been used posttransplant.

Patient Treatment Course

At his first follow-up visit with his PCP, our patient was noted to be newly obese and hypertensive. Routine exercise (specifically 150 minutes per week) and dietary modifications (incorporation of the Mediterranean diet) were recommended to improve his metabolic risk factors. He was advised to purchase a home blood pressure cuff and monitor his blood pressures daily. He was also recommended to monitor his sodium intake and to start amlodipine 5 mg daily if his blood pressure remained elevated. Because of his metabolic risk factors, he was screened for dyslipidemia and DM with a lipid panel and hemoglobin A1c, respectively, and a basic metabolic panel to assess his kidney function. His kidney function was normal; however, his hemoglobin A1c was 6.3%, and his 10-year ASCVD risk based on his demographics, blood pressure, and lipid panel was 12%. He was started on aspirin 81 mg daily and pravastatin 40 mg daily for primary prevention of ASCVD and dyslipidemia, respectively. His continued alcohol abstinence was encouraged. Annual dermatology exam, sun protection, and annual ENT exams to begin 1 year after transplant were discussed.

Two weeks later, the patient reports general malaise of 1 week duration which is not improving. He denies any other symptoms. No new medications or supplements were started and he denies alcohol relapse. An urgent clinic appointment was made later that day. His vital signs are remarkable for a heart rate of 95 and blood pressure of 160/95. His physical exam is normal except he appears fatigued. Labs show an aspartate aminotransferase (AST) of 230 U/L and an alanine aminotransferase (ALT) level of 290 U/L; the rest of his liver chemistry tests, his complete blood count (CBC) and basic metabolic panel (BMP), and his international normalized ratio (INR) are normal.

Question 4. What is the differential diagnosis for and approach to abnormal liver chemistry tests in the LT patient?

Abnormal liver chemistry tests in a LT patient could be due to a variety of causes and should be evaluated urgently. The differential diagnosis is broad, and much like abnormal liver chemistry tests in any patient, the degree of derangement and whether the abnormality is primarily hepatocellular or cholestatic offer clues to the diagnosis. Furthermore, the time from LT is important as specific complications are more likely to occur at certain times in the peri- or posttransplant period.

The best way to approach abnormal liver chemistry tests in the LT patient is to organize the differential diagnosis into the general categories of disease states that can cause these abnormal tests (Table 19.5). Categories for the LT patient should include infection, rejection, vascular abnormalities, biliary abnormalities, drug-induced liver injury, and recurrent liver disease.

Infection is one of the most common causes of liver chemistry abnormalities and morbidity and mortality post-LT. Multiple studies show infections occurring post-LT at rates as high as 64–68%, with bacterial and then viral or fungal organisms being the most common infectious microbes. Most infections happen

Table 19.5 Differential diagnosis for abnormal liver chemistry tests post-OLT

Category	Etiologies	Most common time of onset
Infection	Bacterial, viral, fungal	Perioperatively, decreases substantially 3 months after LT
Rejection	Acute, chronic	Acute: within 3 months of LT Chronic: within 1 year of LT
Vascular abnormality	Early or late hepatic artery thrombosis, portal vein thrombosis, Budd-Chiari syndrome, ischemic hepatopathy	Early HAT: within 1 month of LT Late HAT: >1 month from LT PVT: perioperatively B-CS: perioperatively IH: depending on clinical status
Biliary abnormality	Biliary leaks, anastomotic or non-anastomotic biliary stricture, bile casts, sludge, stones	Biliary leaks: perioperatively and within 3 months of LT AS: within 1 year of LT NAS: within 6 months of LT Bile casts: within 1 year of LT Bile sludge: within 1 year of LT Biliary stones: after 1 year from LT
Drug-induced liver injury	Dependent on medications/supplements taken	Depending on time of ingestion or administration
Recurrent liver disease	NAFLD, alcohol-related liver disease, hepatitis C virus, hepatitis B virus, autoimmune hepatitis, primary biliary cirrhosis, primary sclerosing cholangitis	Varies per disease according to individual, lifestyle, and modifiable risk factors

LT liver transplantation, *HAT* hepatic artery thrombosis, *PVT* portal vein thrombosis, *B-CS* Budd-Chiari syndrome, *IH* ischemic hepatopathy, *AS* anastomotic stricture, *NAS* non-anastomotic stricture, *NAFLD* nonalcoholic fatty liver disease perioperatively, and the incidence of infection decreases abruptly 3 months post-LT, with one series showing two-thirds of infections occurring within the first 100 days of LT. This large proportion of infections early in the post-LT period is likely secondary to contamination within the abdomen, iatrogenic causes such as indwelling urinary and vascular catheters, and complexity of the surgery. Rates of infections have decreased, however, due to the use of the prophylactic antimicrobials mentioned above, improved surgical techniques, and more modest use of immunosuppression.

A thorough history and physical in all LT patients presenting with abnormal liver chemistry tests should be done, with special attention paid to infectious symptoms and signs. A general infectious workup should be done in all patients with any concern for infection, including urine culture, bacterial and fungal blood cultures, and a chest radiograph. Viral testing, including for CMV, EBV, parvovirus, VZV, and HSV, should be considered in all patients. Further workup, including imaging, should be tailored to the patient's symptoms. One study showed that the most frequent infection 2–6 months post-LT was *Enterococcus* related to biliary tract infection. Broad-spectrum antibiotics should be started if the patient appears systemically ill or is hemodynamically unstable until culture results return. LT patients in whom a fungal infection (typically *Candida* or *Aspergillus*) is suspected should be started on antifungal therapy in consultation with an infectious disease specialist.

The fact that our patient does not have a fever does not rule out infection. Fever is not a reliable indicator of infection post-LT. In one study, 40% of patients who had an infection were not febrile, and fevers have also been associated with noninfectious causes post-LT, including medication-induced, malignancy, transfusions, and rejection. Given his weakness, mild tachycardia, and abnormal labs, he should be admitted to the hospital and undergo an appropriate infectious workup as described above.

Acute cellular rejection (ACR) can occur at any time posttransplant but is often diagnosed within the first 3 months post-LT. About 15% of LT patients are diagnosed with ACR. Patient presentation varies, but most are asymptomatic, with routine labs notable for liver chemistry abnormalities. The diagnosis is made by liver biopsy, which shows the classic triad of portal inflammation, endotheliitis, and bile duct injury. Treatment typically involves pulse-dose intravenous steroid therapy with an oral steroid taper, in addition to increasing the patient's existing immunosuppression.

Chronic rejection has become more uncommon in the era of improved immunosuppression, with previous rates of 10% at 5 years post-LT now decreasing to an incidence of less than 5%. Chronic rejection can occur without episodes of ACR or after one or multiple episodes of acute rejection. An elevation in alkaline phosphatase or gamma-glutamyl transpeptidase, due to bile duct injury, is an early indicator that chronic rejection may be occurring. Liver biopsy is needed for diagnosis, and it shows bile duct atrophy in the majority of bile ducts and/or >50% bile duct loss within portal tracts as well as foam cell obliterative arteriopathy. Similarly to acute rejection, treatment consists of increasing the immunosuppression regimen.

Our patient's compliance with his tacrolimus should be assessed, and tacrolimus serum trough levels should be checked for confirmation. Non-compliance and a low tacrolimus level would make a diagnosis of ACR likely, although liver biopsy would be needed for confirmation.

Vascular complications that give rise to liver chemistry abnormalities are rare but are often due to hepatic artery thrombosis, portal vein thrombosis, Budd-Chiari syndrome, or ischemic hepatopathy. Hepatic artery thrombosis (HAT) can be categorized as either early (within 1 month of LT) or late (typically defined as 1–12 months post-LT). Early HAT presents with worsening liver function, and treatment consists of revascularization or often re-transplant. Delayed HAT is more uncommon than early HAT and can be asymptomatic or associated with cholangitis, intra-abdominal abscesses, or biliary leaks. It is treated similarly to early HAT. The most effective means of diagnosis is imaging, either using ultrasound with Doppler, computed tomography (CT), or magnetic resonance imaging (MRI). Similarly, Budd-Chiari syndrome and portal vein thrombosis (PVT) are diagnosed with ultrasound, CT, or MRI, and early manifestations of both can be an asymptomatic patient with mild to moderate elevations in their liver chemistry tests. Ischemic hepatopathy is typically diagnosed in a hemodynamically unstable patient suffering from hypovolemic, hemorrhagic, cardiogenic, or septic shock, and ALT and AST levels are often in the thousand range, while the bilirubin is typically less than 3 mg/dL, and alkaline phosphatase is normal or only mildly elevated.

Although a vascular etiology of our patient's illness is less likely, he should be screened with an abdominal ultrasound with Doppler to rule out HAT, PVT, and Budd-Chiari.

Biliary complications associated with liver transplantation include bile leaks, biliary strictures, and bile casts, sludge, or stones. Biliary disease can present early or late after LT and can be associated with significant morbidity and mortality. Most cases of bile leaks are diagnosed perioperatively or within 1–3 months post-LT, with incidence rates initially reported as high as 19% although more recently rates are reported as 5–7%. Bile leaks can occur at the site of the biliary anastomosis or elsewhere, and patients can be asymptomatic or present with signs of cholestasis and cholangitis (33). The diagnostic gold standard is endoscopic retrograde cholangiopancreatography (ERCP), but patients are often screened first with an ultrasound, with diagnosis often confirmed with magnetic resonance cholangiopancreatography (MRCP). Endoscopic treatment with ERCP-guided sphincterotomy, drainage, and stenting is first-line, although surgical intervention can be considered if endoscopic therapy is unsuccessful.

Biliary strictures are the most common biliary complication after LT, occurring in 4–16% of patients. Mean time to diagnosis is between 5 and 8 months post-LT, although diagnoses can be made years after transplant. Strictures are categorized into anastomotic or non-anastomotic strictures (NAS). Most anastomotic strictures occur within 1 year of LT and are caused by postoperative edema or ischemia. Patients often present with cholestasis and can develop cholangitis, but pain is seldom reported. ERCP or direct cholangiography is the diagnostic gold standard, but MRCP is the best noninvasive test; abdominal ultrasound has a poor diagnostic sensitivity. The majority of patients are treated endoscopically with balloon dilation and stenting, although percutaneous cholangiography (PTC) and surgery remain treatment options. Non-anastomotic strictures can be caused by HAT, ischemia, or rejection. Most NAS present within 6 months of LT and similarly to patients with anastomotic strictures, with cholestatic labs and occasionally cholangitis. Diagnosis and treatment for NAS is the same as for anastomotic strictures, although endoscopic therapy is typically less successful for NAS.

Bile casts, sludge, and stones are often associated with biliary complications post-LT, particularly strictures. Stones and sludge have a prevalence of 5.7%, and cast incidence ranges between 1.6% and 18%. Casts and sludge usually occur within 1 year of LT, while stones typically present after 1 year. Like other biliary complications, both cholestasis and cholangitis can be present, and an ultrasound can be used for diagnosis. Sludge and stones can be treated with ursodeoxycholic acid, although with limited success. Success rates of 90–100% are reported when ERCP is employed. ERCP is less successful for casts, and occasionally surgery is necessary.

Since our patient does not appear infected or have labs suggestive of cholestasis, biliary complications appear to be less likely. A low threshold for more comprehensive imaging such as MRCP should be employed if he develops cholestasis or signs of cholangitis.

Drug-induced liver injury (DILI) is a common cause of liver chemistry abnormalities. A thorough investigation of all prescription and non-prescription medications as well as herbals and supplements should be undertaken. Our patient denies any new medications or supplements. His current medications are unlikely contributing to his transaminitis. Trimethoprim-sulfamethoxazole can cause a cholestatic or mixed cholestatic-hepatocellular injury. Valganciclovir and tacrolimus are not typically associated with clinically significant DILI.

Recurrent liver disease can be a cause of abnormal liver chemistry tests in the LT patient. The most common primary liver diseases that can recur include NAFLD, alcohol-related liver disease, viral hepatitides such HCV or hepatitis B virus, autoimmune hepatitis, primary biliary cirrhosis, and primary sclerosing cholangitis. Alpha-1-antitrypsin deficiency, Wilson's disease, DILI (once the drug is withdrawn), and congenital anomalies are cured with a liver transplant. Our patient's transaminitis is not consistent with alcohol-induced liver injury, and he denies alcohol recidivism. A serum alcohol level should be drawn in any patient with a pertinent history.

Patient Treatment Course (Continued)

The patient was admitted to the hospital and underwent the infectious workup described above. Upon further questioning, he reported occasionally forgetting to take his evening dose of tacrolimus. The following day, his AST and ALT were 250 U/L and 320 U/L, respectively, and his alkaline phosphatase and bilirubin remained normal. His tacrolimus level was 4 ng/mL, less than his goal of 6–8 ng/mL. His liver ultrasound with Doppler was unremarkable, and his infectious workup returned completely negative. He underwent liver biopsy which confirmed a diagnosis of moderate acute cellular rejection. He was started on

IV corticosteroids, with improvement in his transaminases and clinical symptoms. He was instructed on compliance with his tacrolimus, his dosage was increased, and he was discharged on an oral corticosteroid taper.

Conclusions

As outcomes and survival continue to improve for liver transplant recipients, it is imperative that clinicians focus on the care of LT patients in the long term. LT patients are at greater risk for a variety of chronic diseases, particularly the metabolic syndrome, chronic kidney disease, cardiovascular disease, and certain malignancies. LT patients should be screened more intensely for these conditions and treated aggressively. Immunosuppression and antimicrobial prophylaxis are cornerstones of post-LT care. Ensuring patient compliance and physician awareness of side effect profiles are paramount to prevent complications post-LT. Liver chemistry abnormalities are common post-LT and can be caused by infections, rejection, vascular or biliary disease, medications or drugs, and recurrent liver disease.

Further Reading

1. Banff Working Group. Liver biopsy interpretation for causes of late liver allograft dysfunction. Hepatology. 2006;44(2):489–501. https://doi.org/10.1002/hep.21280.
2. Cheung A, Levitsky J. Follow-up of the post-liver transplantation patient. Clin Liver Dis. 2017;21(4):793–813. https://doi.org/10.1016/j.cld.2017.06.006.
3. Demetris AJ, Murase N, Lee RG, et al. Chronic rejection. A general overview of histopathology and pathophysiology with emphasis on liver, heart and intestinal allografts. Ann Transplant. 1997;2(2):27–44.

4. Liu LU, Schiano TD. Long-term care of the liver transplant recipient. Clin Liver Dis. 2007;11(2):397–416. https://doi.org/10.1016/j.cld.2007.04.003.
5. Marino FYCNSTGMMWIR. Fever in liver transplant recipients: changing spectrum of etiologic agents. Clin Infect Dis. 1998;26(1):59–65.
6. Pillai AA. Management of de novo malignancies after liver transplantation. Transplant Rev. 2015;29(1):38–41. https://doi.org/10.1016/j.trre.2014.11.002.
7. Verdonk RC, Buis CI, Porte RJ, Haagsma EB. Biliary complications after liver transplantation: a review. Scand J Gastroenterol Suppl. 2006;243:89–101. https://doi.org/10.1080/00365520600664375.
8. Watt KDS, Charlton MR. Metabolic syndrome and liver transplantation: a review and guide to management. J Hepatol. 2010;53(1):199–206. https://doi.org/10.1016/j.jhep.2010.01.040.

Chapter 20
Reactivation of Hepatitis B

Perica Davitkov and Yngve Falck-Ytter

Introduction

Hepatitis B (HBV) is one of the most common viral infections of the liver worldwide. There are more than two billion people that have been infected, four million acute cases per year, and one million deaths per year. Out of those, 350–400 million are chronic carriers, and 25% of carriers die from chronic hepatitis, cirrhosis, or liver cancer.

HBV reactivation (HBVr) refers to either de novo detection of HBV-DNA, seroreversion (e.g., from negative HBsAg to positive), or more than a tenfold increase in HBV-DNA level compared to baseline, which could lead to a hepatitis flare characterized as a two- to threefold elevation of ALT in a patient with previously inactive or resolved HBV. HBVr can lead to a fatal outcome in 4–60% of cases.

In this chapter, we describe a case of HBVr in an asymptomatic patient undergoing chemotherapy. We discuss screening

P. Davitkov · Y. Falck-Ytter (✉)
Louis Stokes VA Medical Center, Cleveland, OH, USA

Case Western Reserve University, Cleveland, OH, USA

Digestive Health Institute, University Hospitals Cleveland Medical Center, Cleveland, OH, USA
e-mail: Yngve.Falck-Ytter@case.edu

© Springer Nature Switzerland AG 2019
S. M. Cohen, P. Davitkov (eds.), *Liver Disease*,
https://doi.org/10.1007/978-3-319-98506-0_20

strategies, serologic testing, risk of reactivation, and preventive treatment options.

Clinical Case Scenario

A 29-year-old Albanian male was referred to hepatology clinic for evaluation of elevated liver function tests (LFTs). On presentation he denies any specific complaints. He has no nausea, vomiting, diarrhea, current skin rash, abdominal pain, or jaundice. He has a history of beta thalassemia major, and he recently underwent unrelated donor peripheral blood stem cell transplant which was successful. Just prior to his transplant, he had a splenectomy in an effort to reduce hypersplenism and was given a short course of rituximab (8 weeks prior to his current clinic visit). He is currently not on any prescribed drugs and takes no herbal products or over-the-counter medications. Family history reveals no known history of liver disease. He denies alcohol, tobacco, or intravenous drugs. He does have two tattoos and received multiple blood transfusions in the past. He denies any foreign travel for the last few years. He is in a long-term monogamous relationship with his girlfriend. She has not had any jaundice or known liver disease. Physical examination reveals no stigmata of chronic liver disease. Routine labs reveal WBC 13.1, Hgb 13.6, platelets 253, ferritin 11,325 micrograms/L, creatinine 0.62 mg/dL, glucose 92 mg/dL, protein 7.5 g/dL, albumin 3.7 g/dL, alkaline phosphatase 203 U/L, bilirubin 0.4 mg/dL, AST 557 U/L, ALT 1275 U/L, and INR 1.0. Furthermore, HCV is negative, hepatitis A IgM negative, hepatitis B core IgM (anti-HBc IgM) positive, and hepatitis B surface antigen (HBsAg) positive. Lab data from 1 year prior to his presentation revealed hepatitis B surface antigen negative, hepatitis B surface antibody positive (anti-HBs), hepatitis B core IgM negative, hepatitis B core antibody total positive (anti-HBc total), and hepatitis B DNA (HBV-DNA) negative.

Questions

1. What additional serologic testing in regard to HBV will help us understand who might reactivate?
2. With regard to the risk of reactivation due to immunosuppression, is this patient at low-, moderate-, or high-risk?
3. What are the current screening guidelines for HBV in patients who will be undergoing immunosuppressive therapy?
4. Does the presence of antibody to hepatitis B surface antigen (anti-HBs) confer additional protection against HBVr in this patient?
5. What are the prophylactic treatment options for this patient's HBV, and how long should he be on prophylaxis?
6. What advice should be given to this patient in regard to HBV transmission risk?

Discussion

Question 1: What additional serologic testing in regard to HBV will help us understand who might reactivate?

The patient in the clinical case scenario has suffered a reactivation of HBV. Based on the blood tests from 1 year ago, he has been exposed to hepatitis B in the past and had shown evidence of resolution of this infection. However, he was treated with a very potent immunosuppressant drug (rituximab) that resulted in HBVr. Evidence to support reactivation of hepatitis B is elevation of ALT and AST and a positive HBsAg. To confirm the active infection, HBV-DNA level was ordered. In fact, his HBV-DNA came back very elevated (>8.2 logs IU/mL).

For the evaluation of HBV, serologic markers include HBsAg, anti-HBs, anti-HBc total, anti-HBc IgM, hepatitis B e antigen

(HBeAg), hepatitis B e antibody (anti-HBe), and HBV-DNA. The serologic markers typically are used to differentiate between acute, resolving, chronic infection and reactivation. Interpretation of the serologic markers for HBV infection is presented in Table 20.1. Table 20.2 describes how to differentiate between the inactive carrier state, resolved state, and reactivation.

Table 20.1 Interpretation of the serologic markers for HBV infection

	HBsAg	Anti-HBc total	Anti-HBc IgM	Anti-HBs	What it means
A	−	−	−	−	Never exposed
B	−	−	−	+	Vaccinated
C[a]	−	+	−	+	Immunity (past infection)
D[a]	+	+	+	−	Acute HBV
E[a]	+	+	−	−	Chronic HBV
F	+	+	+/−	−	HBV reactivation

[a]Patients with serologic markers as described at rows C, D, and E are all at risk for reactivation

Table 20.2 Differentiating inactive carrier state, resolved infection, and reactivation

	Inactive carrier	Resolved infection	Reactivation
HBsAg	+	−	+
HBeAg	−	−	+/−
Anti-HBc total	+	+	+
ALT/AST	Normal	Normal	Elevated or fluctuating
HBV-DNA	<2000 IU/mL	Undetectable	Moderate or fluctuating (>2000 IU/mL)
Histology	Absence of hepatitis, minimal fibrosis	Absence of hepatitis, no fibrosis	Variable fibrosis

Question 2: With regard to the risk of reactivation due to immunosuppression, is this patient at low-, moderate-, or high-risk?

The risk of HBVr among patients presenting with different serological patterns that indicate either ongoing or recovered HBV infection (HBsAg positive/anti-HBc positive or HBsAg negative/anti-HBc positive, respectively) varies depending on the type of immunosuppression. In order to determine who will benefit from prophylactic antiviral treatment, immuno-suppressants have been categorized into low-, moderate-, or high-risk groups based on estimates of likelihood of reactivation. The high-risk group is defined by anticipated incidence of HBVr in >10%. The moderate-risk group is defined by anticipated incidence of HBVr in 1% to 10% of cases. The low-risk group is defined by anticipated incidence of HBVr in <1% of cases.

Tables 20.3, 20.4, and 20.5 describe the risk of HBVr in patients with ongoing (*HBsAg + anti-HBc total +*) or recovered (*HBsAg -anti-HBc total +*) HBV infection exposed to different immunosuppressants.

Table 20.3 High-risk group for HBVr (>10%)

	HBsAg + anti-HBc total +	HBsAg - anti-HBc total +
B-cell-depleting agents (*rituximab, ofatumumab*)	30–60%	17%
Anthracycline derivatives (e.g., *doxorubicin/epirubicin*)	15–30%	
Corticosteroids for >4 weeks (*>10 mg prednisone*)	>10%	

Table 20.4 Moderate-risk group for HBVr (1–10%)

	HBsAg + anti-HBc total +	HBsAg – anti-HBc total +
TNF-alpha inhibitors (*etanercept, adalimumab, certolizumab, infliximab*)	1–10%	1%
Other cytokine and integrin inhibitors (*abatacept, ustekinumab, natalizumab, vedolizumab*)	1–10%	1%
Tyrosine kinase inhibitors (*imatinib, nilotinib*)	1–10%	1%
Corticosteroids for >4 weeks	1–10% *Low dose <10 mg*	1–10% *High dose >10 mg*
Anthracycline derivatives (e.g., *doxorubicin/epirubicin*)		1%

Table 20.5 Low-risk group for HBVr (<1%)

	HBsAg + anti-HBc total +	HBsAg – anti-HBc total +
Traditional immunosuppressant agents (*azathioprine, 6-mercaptopurine, methotrexate alone*)	<1%	<1%
Intra-articular corticosteroid	<1%	<1%
Corticosteroids for ≤ 1 week	<1%	<1%
Corticosteroids for >4 weeks		<1% *Low dose <10 mg*

Based on the information from Tables 20.3, 20.4, and 20.5 and the patient's clinical data, our patient was at high-risk for reactivation because he was HBsAg –/HBcAb + and received rituximab. However, he was not given HBV prophylaxis.

Question 3: What are the current screening guidelines for HBV in patients who will be undergoing immunosuppressive therapy?

The benefits of screening include early identification of chronic HBV infection or resolved HBV infection in patients who will be treated with immunosuppressive therapy such that prophylaxis can be used, if appropriate, to minimize the risk of reactivation and associated morbidity and mortality. Thus, the American Gastroenterological Association (AGA) recommends that patients who are at moderate- or high-risk and who are undergoing immunosuppressive therapy should be routinely screened for HBV by ordering HBsAg and anti-HBc, followed by a sensitive HBV-DNA test if positive. In patients that are at low-risk and will be receiving immunosuppressive therapy, the AGA suggests against routine screening for HBV infection.

The patient in our scenario had positive anti-HBc total, and he was going to be treated with rituximab; this puts him at high-risk group that would require screening.

Question 4: Does the presence of antibody to hepatitis B surface antigen (anti-HBs) confer additional protection against HBVr in this patient?

The patient in our case scenario had detectable anti-HBs, and one may think that he would be protected from HBVr. Even though it has been suggested that the presence of anti-HBs may provide additional protection against reactivation, there have been small numbers of cases reported, with positive anti-HBs where HBVr occurred. Thus, the AGA guidelines suggest against using anti-HBs status to guide antiviral prophylaxis for all risk groups.

Question 5: What are the prophylactic treatment options for this patient's HBV, and how long should he be on prophylaxis?

Our patient is at high-risk due to intense immunosuppressive therapy. He should have been started on antiviral prophylaxis.

The AGA recommends antiviral prophylaxis over no prophylaxis for patients at high- and moderate-risk undergoing immunosuppressive drug therapy. The AGA suggests against routinely using antiviral prophylaxis in patients undergoing immunosuppressive drug therapy who are at low-risk for HBVr. Risk groups were discussed above and in Tables 20.3, 20.4, and 20.5.

When a long duration of immunosuppressive treatment is anticipated, tenofovir and entecavir are the preferred HBV antiviral agents because of their safety profile and low potential for developing resistance. If a short duration (<12 months) of therapy is anticipated, then lamivudine or telbivudine may also be considered as options in the setting of undetectable or low baseline serum HBV-DNA levels. Interferon alfa should be avoided in view of the bone marrow suppressive effect.

A randomized controlled trial of entecavir versus lamivudine prophylaxis showed decreased risk of HBVr, HBV flare, and disruption of chemotherapy with the use of entecavir over lamivudine. In addition, antiviral drugs with a high barrier to resistance when compared to lamivudine in established HBV reactivation showed significantly lower viral resistance and failure of virologic response. Thus, the AGA suggests the use of antiviral drugs with a high barrier to resistance (e.g., tenofovir or entecavir) over lamivudine for prophylaxis and treatment in such patients undergoing immunosuppressive drug therapy.

For the high-risk group (>10%) (Table 20.3), prophylactic treatment should be continued for at least 6 months after discontinuation of immunosuppressive therapy (at least 12 months for B-cell-depleting agents). Furthermore, for patients in the moderate-risk group (1–10%) (Table 20.4), treatment should be continued for 6 months after discontinuation of immunosuppressive therapy.

Question 6: What advice should be given to this patient in regard to HBV transmission risk?

Transmission risk for HBV in this patient is similar to a patient with active HBV infection. Transmission for HBV is common. In fact, HBV is 100 times more contagious than HIV. HBV is transmitted through activities that involve percutaneous or mucosal contact with infectious blood or body fluids (semen, saliva). These activities include sex with an infected partner; injection drug use that involves sharing needles, syringes, or drug preparation equipment; birth to an infected mother; contact with blood or open sores of an infected person; needle sticks or sharp instrument exposures; and sharing items such as razors or toothbrushes with an infected person. HBV is usually not spread through food or water, sharing eating utensils, breastfeeding, hugging, kissing, hand holding, coughing, or sneezing.

In our case scenario, the patient's partner should see her primary care physician as soon as possible to discuss testing, vaccination, and possibly even hepatitis B immune globulin (HBIg) administration.

Patient Treatment Course

As discussed before, at the initial visit, there was a high concern about HBVr given the fact that HBsAg became positive. For that reason, HBV-DNA was sent and the patient was started on entecavir 1 mg daily. In fact, his HBV-DNA was found to be very elevated (>8.2 logs IU/mL). He was monitored closely with LFTs and HBV-DNA levels.

Just a few months after the initiation of antiviral therapy, his LFTs normalized, and his HBV-DNA became undetectable. Liver biopsy was performed to assess the stage of his liver disease. The biopsy showed periportal fibrosis. The plan is to monitor LFTs and HBV-DNA more frequently, but once stable he will have annual check of HBsAg and anti-HBs in addition to appropriate hepatocellular carcinoma screening similar to patients with chronic HBV.

Conclusions

HBV reactivation is common with immunosuppression, can be clinically severe, and can result in death from acute liver failure or progressive liver disease and cirrhosis. It is important to screen for HBsAg and anti-HBc in all patients before undergoing cancer chemotherapy, marked immunosuppressive treatment, or solid organ or bone marrow transplantation. HBVr prophylaxis is highly effective and recommended in moderate- and high-risk populations. HBV prophylaxis should be continued for at least 6 months after stopping most chemotherapy and at least 12 months after completing B-cell-depleting agents. Consider long-term HBV prophylaxis with an antiviral with a high barrier to resistance (tenofovir or entecavir).

Disclosure   The authors of this manuscript have no conflicts of interest to disclose.

Further Reading

1. CDC guidelines on HBV. https://www.cdc.gov/hepatitis/hbv/hbvfaq. htm#treatment
2. Huang H, Li XY, Li HR, et al. Preventing hepatitis B reactivation in HBsAg-positive patients with untreated diffuse large B-cell lymphoma with R-CHOP chemotherapy: a prospective study to compare entecavir and lamivudine. J Clin Oncol. 2013;31:8503–3.
3. Martin P, Lau DT, Nguyen MH, et al. A treatment algorithm for the management of chronic hepatitis B virus infection in the United States: 2015 update. Clin Gastroenterol Hepatol. 2015;13:2071–87.
4. Perrillo RP, Gish R, Falck-Ytter Y. American Gastroenterological Association Institute technical review on prevention and treatment of hepatitis B virus reactivation during immunosuppressive drug therapy. Gastroenterology. 2015 Jan;148(1):221–44.
5. Reddy KR, Beavers KL, Hammond SP, Lim JK, Falck-Ytter YT, AGA Institute. American Gastroenterological Association Institute guideline on the prevention and treatment of hepatitis B virus reactivation during immunosuppressive drug therapy. Gastroenterology. 2015 Jan;148(1):215–9.
6. Weinbaum CM, Williams I, Mast EE, et al. Recommendations for identification and public health management of persons with chronic hepatitis B virus infection. MMWR Recomm Rep. *2008;57(RR-8):1–20.*

Chapter 21
Surgery in the Patient with Chronic Liver Disease

Jason J. Cano and Stephen C. Pappas

Introduction

Patients with chronic liver disease including cirrhosis are now being offered surgery more than ever before. Surgical risk in the patient with cirrhosis is complex and depends on multiple factors including severity of liver disease, surgical procedure, urgency of the procedure, type of sedation, and presence of comorbid conditions. However, there are currently no rigorous evidence-based guidelines to aid the clinician in the management of the patient with chronic liver disease undergoing surgery. Many studies regarding the subject are small, retrospective, and outdated. In this chapter, we outline the principles involved in the management of patients with chronic liver disease undergoing surgery.

J. J. Cano · S. C. Pappas (✉)
Division of Gastroenterology and Hepatology, Baylor College
of Medicine, Houston, TX, USA
e-mail: scpappas@bcm.edu

© Springer Nature Switzerland AG 2019
S. M. Cohen, P. Davitkov (eds.), *Liver Disease*,
https://doi.org/10.1007/978-3-319-98506-0_21

Clinical Case Scenario

A 34-year-old woman with decompensated, alcohol-induced cirrhosis is referred by her gynecologist for an opinion regarding elective removal of an ovarian cystic lesion with characteristics worrisome for malignancy. Hepatic decompensation is characterized by a history of ascites, currently controlled by a low sodium diet in combination with low-dose furosemide and Aldactone. She has been abstinent from alcohol for the past 7 months and has gained some weight from improved nutrition. Physical examination reveals no evidence of hepatic encephalopathy, a non-distended abdomen, and resolution of spider angiomata observed on prior examinations. She has had a recent esophagogastroduodenoscopy that revealed small esophageal varices without high-risk stigmata. She is up to date with hepatocellular carcinoma screening. Her labs are notable for a serum sodium of 137 mmol/L, albumin of 3.8 g/dL, creatinine of 0.97 mg/dL, ALT of 23 U/L, AST of 52 U/L, alkaline phosphatase of 152 IU/L, total bilirubin of 1.2 mg/dL, hemoglobin of 13 g/dL, platelets of 95,000 per liter, and INR of 1.1. Her Model for End-Stage Liver Disease (MELD) score is 11, and she has Child-Turcotte-Pugh (CTP) class B cirrhosis.

Questions

1. What preoperative assessment and risk stratification should be performed on this patient prior to surgery?
2. Are there surgical risks specific to patients with cirrhosis?
3. Does the type of surgery have an impact on outcomes?
4. Should this patient have a transjugular intrahepatic portosystemic shunt (TIPS) prior to surgery?
5. How should this patient be managed during and after surgery?

Question 1. What preoperative assessment and risk stratification should be performed on this patient prior to surgery?

History and physical examination should be the initial assessment to evaluate the severity of liver disease and degree of portal hypertension. Focus should be paid to determine if there is a history of decompensation of liver disease including a history of altered mental status, gastrointestinal bleeding, and increased abdominal girth. Additionally, nutrition status should be evaluated to assess for malnutrition.

A complete blood count, comprehensive metabolic panel, INR, prothrombin time (PT), and partial thromboplastic time (PTT) should be obtained as part of a thorough preoperative risk assessment.

The presence of thrombocytopenia, splenomegaly, varices, ascites, and a hepatic venous pressure gradient greater than 10 mmHg are features that suggest clinically significant portal hypertension.

Multiple variables have been assessed to determine operative risk stratification for patients with cirrhosis undergoing surgery. However, traditional preoperative risk assessment tools such as the American Society of Anesthesiologists (ASA) physical classification do not take into account risks specific to patients with chronic liver disease such as portal hypertension and poor nutritional status.

Currently, perioperative risk assessment in patients with cirrhosis undergoing surgery is most commonly assessed by the CTP class and MELD score. Several studies have shown that the degree of hepatic decompensation as assessed by CTP and MELD is the most important factor that determines perioperative morbidity and mortality.

The CTP class is based on the patient's serum bilirubin, serum albumin, INR, degree of ascites, and presence of hepatic encephalopathy. The CTP has been validated in small retrospective studies with general surgery mortality rates as high as 10% for CTP class A, 30% for CTP class B, and 76–82% for those with CTP class C cirrhosis. More recent studies have suggested a much reduced mortality rate of 2% for those patients with CTP class A cirrhosis and 12% for CTP classes B and C cirrhosis, suggesting current surgical techniques and medical monitoring have improved significantly since these initial studies. Although the CTP is easily calculated and commonly used, it has multiple subjective components that may result in clinicians under- or overestimating liver function as variables are categorized using arbitrary cutoff values.

Unlike the CTP classification, the MELD score was not originally developed for surgical risk assessment. However, it has been shown to be a good predictor of 30-day, 90-day, and long-term postoperative mortality. The MELD score is based on objective data including the patient's serum bilirubin, serum creatinine, and INR; hence, it is more objective and reproducible. In prior studies, for every MELD score point increase above 8, there was a 14% increase in the relative risk of mortality in the first 30 to 90 days post-surgery. Median survival after surgery based on the MELD score has been shown to be as follows: MELD 0–7, 4.8 years; MELD 8–11, 3.4 years; MELD 12–15, 1.6 years; MELD 16–20, 64 days; MELD 21–25, 23 days; and MELD >26, 14 days.

The CTP and MELD scores are not mutually exclusive, and it is advised that both assessments be used to guide clinical management, noting that the MELD score may be more precise in those patients with decompensated cirrhosis.

Teh et al., in the largest retrospective study of predictors of perioperative mortality in patients with cirrhosis, evaluated over 700 cirrhotic patients undergoing orthopedic, cardiac, and gastrointestinal surgeries. Results showed that in addition to the MELD score, the patient's age and ASA class were statistically significant and independent predictors of mortality. Age >70 added the equivalent of 3 MELD points to the mortality rate. Additionally, ASA class was the strongest predictor of 7-day mortality rate; an ASA class of IV added the equivalent of 5.5 MELD points to a patient's morality rate. Although only ten patients with an ASA score of V underwent surgery, 100% died. This study supported the development of the Mayo Clinic Postoperative Mortality Risk in Patients with Cirrhosis Model which can be used to estimate 7-day, 30-day, 90-day, 1-year, and 5-year mortality rates after surgery. A web-based calculator is available at http://www.mayoclinic.org/meld/mayomodel9.html.

Question 2. Are there surgical risks specific to patients with cirrhosis?

In patients with cirrhosis who are to undergo surgery, special attention should be paid to the patient's mental status, nutritional status, coagulation status, electrolytes, ascites, esophageal varices, and alcohol use.

Hepatic Encephalopathy A careful assessment for covert hepatic encephalopathy should be performed as surgery can precipitate overt hepatic encephalopathy which can significantly impair postoperative care.

Esophageal Varices Variceal hemorrhage is a common fear for practitioners who care for patients with cirrhosis. Surgery does not put a patient with cirrhosis and esophageal varices at an increased risk of variceal hemorrhage per se; however, fluid overload can result in increased portal hypertension and thus precipitate a bleed. Patients with cirrhosis should have appropriate variceal screening based on the degree of liver disease prior to surgery. Those patients with small esophageal varices in conjunction with CTP class B or C cirrhosis or large varices regardless of

CTP class require prophylaxis with nonselective beta-blockers such as propranolol or nadolol.

Ascites   In those patients with ascites, a low sodium diet (2 grams per day) and diuretics at appropriate doses should be continued to prevent accumulation of ascites.

Coagulopathy   Patients with cirrhosis and portal hypertension often have an elevated PT, PTT, and INR. Coagulopathy in cirrhosis results from a complex process affecting levels of both procoagulants and anticoagulants. An elevated INR in a patient with cirrhosis is not equivalent to an elevated bleeding risk. However, while noting that the coagulopathy of liver synthetic impairment cannot be corrected with vitamin K supplementation, for an elective surgery, vitamin K should be administered in the event malabsorption is contributing to coagulopathy. Additionally, thrombocytopenia is also commonly present due to hypersplenism and thrombopoietin deficiency. A platelet transfusion goal of greater than 50,000 and greater than 100,000 has been traditionally recommended for those undergoing moderate-and high-risk surgery, respectively. In May 2018, the US Food and Drug Administration approved avatrombopag to treat thrombocytopenia in adults with chronic liver disease who are scheduled to undergo medical or dental procedures. Avatrombopag is an oral thrombopoietin receptor agonist given 5 days prior to a scheduled procedure in those patients that would typically require platelet transfusions. Patient who received avatrombopag had higher platelet counts and required less platelet transfusions and less rescue therapy for up to 7 days following their procedure. If available, thromboelastography, which assesses all phases of clot formation and lysis, should be obtained near the time of surgery.

Malnutrition   Malnutrition is a common finding in patients with chronic liver disease. Several factors contribute to malnutrition including decreased food intake due to abdominal distention from ascites, impaired absorption of nutrients, and increased catabolism. Malnutrition is an independent risk factor for mortality in patients with cirrhosis. Assessment of nutrition can be challenging, but efforts should be made to assess lean body mass, muscle function, and serum albumin. Trace element and vitamin deficiencies (including zinc, magnesium, copper, folate, and vitamin B12) are often observed. If discovered, these deficiencies should be corrected as they can impair wound healing and increase the risk of infectious complications. Preoperative assessment by a dietitian should be performed where available.

Alcohol Use In those patients with a history of heavy alcohol use, a period of alcohol abstinence should be encouraged prior to any elective surgery.

Question 3. Does the type of surgery have an impact on outcomes?

The type of surgery has significant implications for mortality and morbidity in the cirrhotic patient. It is important to understand, however, that many studies on surgical risk do not include patients with advanced liver disease; patients with CTP classes B and C cirrhosis are commonly not offered surgery.

Elective surgery should be planned whenever possible to ensure medical optimization prior to surgery. CTP class A patients can undergo most elective surgical procedures with a reasonable safety profile. Those patients with CTP class C and MELD above 15 should generally avoid elective surgical procedures unless absolutely required.

Generally accepted contraindications to elective surgery in patients with chronic liver disease are included in Table 21.1.

Table 21.1 Contraindications to elective surgery in patients with cirrhosis

1. ASA class V
2. Acute renal failure including hepatorenal syndrome
3. Acute alcoholic hepatitis
4. Severe coagulopathy (treatment refractory)
5. Significant associated or coincidental cardiac dysfunction (including cirrhotic cardiomyopathy)
6. Hypoxemia
7. Acute viral hepatitis
8. Acute liver failure

Emergent surgeries should be performed without delay, but with the understanding that those with decompensated cirrhosis frequently have poor surgical outcomes and increased duration of hospitalization. Emergency surgical procedures have been associated with a mortality of up to 57%.

Consideration should be given to having surgery performed at a liver transplant center with specialized intensive care facilities; improved outcomes have been demonstrated in these settings. Preoperative assessment for possible liver transplantation in the event of postsurgical severe decompensation should be considered in selected patients for whom transplantation is available and appropriate.

Gynecological Surgery Data on gynecological surgeries in patients with cirrhosis is limited. Available studies demonstrate higher morbidity and mortality in patients with cirrhosis compared to control patients undergoing hysterectomy and surgery for gynecological cancer.

Hepatic Resection Hepatic resection for hepatocellular carcinoma (HCC) is generally not an indication for surgery in patients with advanced cirrhosis. Patients with cirrhosis require more residual liver volume than a patient with normal liver given the remaining liver is dysfunctional. Patients with HCC, cirrhosis, and MELD ≥ 9 who undergo hepatic resection have a high risk of mortality (approximately 30%). It seems reasonable to propose that patients with cirrhosis and MELD scores of less than 9 may be able to undergo hepatic resection, patients with a MELD score of 9 to 10 should undergo only limited resection or segmentectomy, and patients with a MELD greater than 10 should not undergo hepatic resection due to the high risk of mortality.

Biliary Surgery Patients with cirrhosis are at risk for biliary disease, in particular pigment gallstone formation. A specific concern for surgeons is the formation of varices in the biliary bed. Laparoscopic surgery rather than open abdominal surgery should be performed when possible and is considered acceptable in patients with CTP class A or B cirrhosis or MELD score <18 without significant portal hypertension. In patients with CTP class C, or when emergency surgery is required, cholecystostomy tube placement, rather than a cholecystectomy, should be performed. Endoscopic and percutaneous biliary drainage is always preferable to surgery for biliary obstruction. Although endoscopic sphincterotomy via endoscopic retrograde cholangiopancreatography (ERCP) is associated with increased risk of bleeding in patients with cirrhosis, the risk is low even in those with CTP class C cirrhosis. In patients with coagulopathy or thrombocytopenia, endoscopic papillary balloon dilation is associated with a lower risk of bleeding than sphincterotomy.

Hernia Repair Umbilical hernias are common findings and are of concern in patients with cirrhosis due to increased intra-abdominal pressure from ascites, muscle weakness, and malnutrition. If possible, umbilical hernias should be repaired prior to the development of ascites. If ascites is present, it should be controlled prior to surgery to decrease the risk of wound dehiscence and poor healing. Rupture of an umbilical hernia in the cirrhotic patient is associated with high mortality. Umbilical hernias have been successfully repaired in patients with CTP class C cirrhosis;

however, caution should be used if the patient has a high MELD score or hypoalbuminemia, due to the risk of infectious complications. Optimal medical management of ascites is crucial post-surgery to prevent recurrence of umbilical hernias.

Gastric Surgery Peptic ulcer disease is common in patients with chronic liver disease. If there is concern for peptic ulcer disease, an EGD should be performed to diagnose, risk stratify, and possibly treat. If surgical therapy is required, a laparoscopic approach should be performed, if possible. A mortality rate of about 10% has been observed in those with cirrhosis requiring gastric surgery.

Colorectal Surgery Colorectal surgery in patients with CTP class A cirrhosis is generally considered safe. Overall, colorectal surgery in patients with cirrhosis is associated with a 26% mortality risk and postoperative complications related to stomal or anastomotic leaks.

Cardiac Surgery Cirrhosis is a well-recognized risk factor for mortality after cardiac surgery. The high risk of mortality is related to the hemodynamic changes associated with liver disease rather than the surgery itself. In patients with CTP class A cirrhosis, cardiac surgery, including cardiopulmonary bypass, may be performed safely. However, patients with advanced cirrhosis have a high mortality, ranging from 50% to 80% in those with CTP class B and 100% for CTP class C cirrhosis. One study of 30-day mortality after cardiac surgery showed 9%, 37%, and 52% mortality in CTP classes A, B, and C cirrhosis patients, respectively. MELD score has also been used to predict mortality after cardiac surgery with a score greater than 13 predicting a poor prognosis. Again, consideration should be given to having cardiac surgery performed at a liver transplant center with specialized intensive care facilities.

Question 4. Should this patient have a transjugular intrahepatic portosystemic shunt (TIPS) prior to surgery?

In the largest study involving preoperative TIPS to reduce portal hypertension, 25 patients with a median MELD score of 15 (28% CTP class C) showed a perioperative mortality risk rate of 12% with prophylactic TIPS placement. Placement of a TIPS approximately 4 to 6 weeks before surgery may allow patients to undergo surgery that normally would be contraindicated. TIPS may also be a preoperative consideration in patients with severe or refractory ascites prohibiting surgery. Overall however, data regarding the precise role of TIPS in decreasing operative mortality and morbidity is limited. In individual selected patients, TIPS placement may be appropriate after a careful risk-benefit analysis has been performed.

Question 5. How should this patient be managed during and after surgery?

When possible, an anesthetist and surgeon with experience in managing patients with chronic liver disease should participate in the surgical procedure. During surgery, the cirrhotic liver is increasingly susceptible to hypoxemia and hypotension. In particular, intraoperative fluid management can be difficult. Crystalloid-based intravenous fluids such as normal saline may worsen ascites and edema, but have minimal effect on effective intravascular volume. Instead, volume expanders such as concentrated albumin should be used. In patients with ascites, perioperative antibiotics with gram-negative bacteria coverage should be provided to reduce the risk of bacterial peritonitis from potential bacteremia that may occur during the procedure.

In general, propofol is considered safe in patients with cirrhosis: it is associated with improved induction, sedation efficacy, recovery, and psychometric recovery, without exacerbation of hepatic encephalopathy.

Surgeries are often followed by minor abnormalities in serum liver chemistries that are not clinically significant. However, in patients with chronic liver disease and specifically cirrhosis, surgery can precipitate hepatic decompensation. The type of injury can range from cholestatic to ischemic hepatic injury. Overall, postoperative complications in patients with cirrhosis have been reported in up to 30% of patients.

In the postoperative period, patients should be monitored for the development of ascites, hepatic encephalopathy, infection, renal injury, or hemorrhage. Intractable ascites after abdominal surgery may occur in up to 40% of CTP class B patients, even occurring in up to 5% of CTP class A patients.

Careful attention should be paid to minimize the possibilities of postoperative complications by maintaining a low sodium diet, avoiding excess fluid replacement, preventing constipation, monitoring renal function, and, if analgesics or sedatives are required, minimizing dose and increasing dosage intervals to avoid accumulation. Acetaminophen is not contraindicated but should be used with caution, not exceeding 2 grams per day. Nonsteroidal anti-inflammatory drugs should be avoided.

Additional Clinical Information and Course

The patient was discussed between the gynecologist, the hepatologist, and a liver transplant surgeon. The lesion was felt to be suspicious for malignancy and needed to be resected. The patient was felt to be relatively well compensated with a MELD score of 11 and CTP B. A TIPS was not deemed to be necessary in the absence of ascites or significant varices. No further preoperative testing was performed. She underwent an uneventful resection of the lesion without evidence of hepatic decompensation. Postoperative surgical recovery was relatively uneventful, and she was discharged home on postoperative day 6.

Conclusions

Patients with cirrhosis have a unique physiology that requires specialized evaluation prior to any surgical procedure. Current management is largely based on retrospective data and expert opinion; prospective and true evidence-based data are very limited. Given the significant risk of morbidity and mortality of surgery in the patient with cirrhosis, meticulous preoperative assessment, management, and risk-benefit analysis should be performed by physicians experienced in the management of chronic liver disease.

Further Reading

1. Befeler AS. The safety of intra-abdominal surgery in patients with cirrhosis. Arch Surg. 2005;140(7):650. https://doi.org/10.1001/archsurg.140.7.650.
2. Bhangui P, Laurent A, Amathieu R, Azoulay D. Assessment of risk for non-hepatic surgery in cirrhotic patients. J Hepatol. 2012;57(4):874–84. https://doi.org/10.1016/j.jhep.2012.03.037.
3. Hanje AJ, Patel T. Preoperative evaluation of patients with liver disease. Nat Clin Pract Gastroenterol Hepatol. 2007;4(5):266–76. https://doi.org/10.1038/ncpgasthep0794.
4. Neeff H, Mariaskin D, Spangenberg HC, Hopt UT, Makowiec F. Perioperative mortality after non-hepatic general surgery in patients with liver cirrhosis: an analysis of 138 operations in the 2000s using child and MELD scores. J Gastrointest Surg. 2011;15(1):1–11. https://doi.org/10.1007/s11605-010-1366-9.

 5. Nicoll A. Surgical risk in patients with cirrhosis. J Gastroenterol Hepatol. 2012;27(10):1569–75.https://doi.org/10.1111/j.1440-1746.2012.07205.x.
 6. O'Leary JG, Friedman LS. Predicting surgical risk in patients with cirrhosis: from art to science. Gastroenterology. 2007;132(4):1609–11. https://doi.org/10.1053/j.gastro.2007.03.016.
 7. Teh SH, Nagorney DM, Stevens SR, et al. Risk factors for mortality after surgery in patients with cirrhosis. Gastroenterology. 2007;132(4):1261–9. https://doi.org/10.1053/j.gastro.2007.01.040.
 8. Telem D, Schiano T, Goldstone R, et al. Factors that predict outcome of abdominal operations in patients with advanced cirrhosis. Clin Gastroenterol Hepatol. 2010;8(5):451–7., quiz e58. https://doi.org/10.1016/j.cgh.2009.12.015.
 9. Ziser A, Plevak DJ, Wiesner RH, Rakela J, Offord KP, Brown DL. Morbidity and mortality in cirrhotic patients undergoing anesthesia and surgery. Anesthesiology. 1999;90(1):42–53. https://doi.org/10.1097/00000542-199901000-00008.

Index

© Springer Nature Switzerland AG 2019

S. M. Cohen, P. Davitkov (eds.), *Liver Disease*,

https://doi.org/10.1007/978-3-319-98506-0